EXPLAINING ABNORMAL BEHAVIOR

Also available

The Development of Psychopathology: Nature and Nurture
Bruce F. Pennington

Diagnosing Learning Disorders:
A Neuropsychological Framework, Second Edition
Bruce F. Pennington

Pediatric Neuropsychology:
Research, Theory, and Practice, Second Edition
Edited by Keith Owen Yeates, M. Douglas Ris,
H. Gerry Taylor, and Bruce F. Pennington

EXPLAINING ABNORMAL BEHAVIOR

A Cognitive Neuroscience Perspective

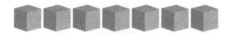

BRUCE F. PENNINGTON

THE GUILFORD PRESS
New York   London

Last digit is print number: 9   8   7   6   5   4   3   2   1

The author has checked with sources believed to be reliable in his efforts
to provide information that is complete and generally in accord with the
standards of practice that are accepted at the time of publication. However,
in view of the possibility of human error or changes in behavioral, mental
health, or medical sciences, neither the author, nor the editor and publisher,
nor any other party who has been involved in the preparation or publication
of this work warrants that the information contained herein is in every
respect accurate or complete, and they are not responsible for any errors or
omissions or the results obtained from the use of such information. Readers
are encouraged to confirm the information contained in this book with other
sources.

Library of Congress Cataloging-in-Publication Data

Pennington, Bruce Franklin, 1946–
    Explaining abnormal behavior : a cognitive neuroscience perspective / Bruce
F. Pennington.
       pages cm
    Includes bibliographical references and index.
    ISBN 978-1-4625-1366-6 (hardcover : alk. paper)
    1. Psychology, Pathological.   2. Mental illness—Etiology.   3. Cognitive
neuroscience.   I. Title.
    RC454.P394 2014
    616.89—dc23
                                                                    2013045526

To the memory of Guy Van Orden

About the Author

Bruce F. Pennington, PhD, is John Evans Professor of Psychology at the University of Denver, where he heads the Developmental Cognitive Neuroscience program. His research focuses on dyslexia, attention-deficit/hyperactivity disorder (ADHD), and autism, with particular interests in using genetic and neuropsychological methods to understand comorbidity among disorders. In addition to being a researcher and research mentor, he is also a child clinical neuropsychologist, and has been active in clinical practice and training throughout his career. Dr. Pennington is a recipient of Research Scientist, MERIT, and Fogarty awards from the National Institutes of Health; the Samuel T. Orton Award from the International Dyslexia Association; and the Emanuel Miller Memorial Lecture from the British Association for Child and Adolescent Mental Health. He is also a Fellow of the American Association for the Advancement of Science and the Association for Psychological Science. He is the author of *Diagnosing Learning Disorders, Second Edition*, and coeditor (with Keith Owen Yeates et al.) of *Pediatric Neuropsychology, Second Edition*.

Preface

Abnormal behavior is fascinating, particularly on an individual level—how is it possible for a person to see and hear things that aren't there? Why does another person claim her parent is an imposter, or a third person deny that his left leg belongs to him? However, abnormal behaviors can also be intriguing because of the information they offer about how *typical* people function. Why do most people recognize their parents day after day, and how do we know which hand is ours? Observations of abnormal behaviors pose mysteries to be solved and can profoundly challenge our beliefs about the self and our control over our own behavior. We will consider these and other examples of abnormal behavior and examine their implications for how our selves actually work.

For nearly all of human history, the explanations for abnormal behavior have been woefully inadequate. In everyday or folk psychology, we typically explain behavior with reference to an actor's beliefs and desires and we assume the actor is rational. When an actor's behavior deviates from the rational norm, folk psychology offers two options for explanation: (1) the actor's behavior actually makes sense in a broader context or (2) the behavior doesn't make sense and is therefore "crazy." The broader context might include the actor's childhood or previous social interactions, for example. The second option is not really an explanation because it just asserts that the behavior is unexplainable. With increasing exposure to neuroscience research, everyday or popular psychology has a new explanatory option for abnormal behavior: "there is something wrong with the actor's brain." For example, the popular media reported that John Hinckley shot President Ronald Reagan because Hinckley was schizophrenic, and what made this explanation convincing was that a structural magnetic resonance imaging scan revealed that Hinckley had enlarged ventricles, which are associated with schizophrenia (and many other disorders, as well). So, for better *and* worse, explanations of abnormal behavior in terms of the brain are being assimilated into everyday psychology. This book is about our current research-based brain explanations for abnormal behavior, including both their scope *and* limits. The goals of this book are to explain cognitive neuroscience models for abnormal behavior so that they are easily understood by nonspecialists and to review how adequate these models are. What is novel about this book is that it attempts to apply the same set of models to virtually the entire domain of abnormal behavior across three different kinds of disorders: neurological disorders, psychiatric disorders, and neurodevelopmental disorders.

Historically, neurologists have focused on syndromes with an identifiable etiology, such as an acquired lesion (e.g., aphasia) or a genetic syndrome (e.g., Huntington's disease) or an identifiable pathophysiology (e.g., plaques and neurofibrillary tangles in Alzheimer's disease). Psychiatrists have focused on behaviorally defined disorders that lack a clear etiology or pathophysiology (e.g., major depression or schizophrenia). Neurodevelopmental disorders overlap with both of the previous two categories because some neurodevelopmental disorders are defined etiologically (e.g., early-treated phenylketonuria [PKU] and Down syndrome) and some are defined behaviorally (e.g., dyslexia and autism), but all are considered to arise from changes in brain development. It is increasingly recognized that most psychiatric disorders are neurodevelopmental disorders as well, because their precursors are evident in childhood and are thought to arise from changes in brain development. A developmental perspective is also important for studying neurological disorders, even acquired ones, because the behavioral manifestations of brain lesions depend crucially on the point in development at which they are acquired. In genetically influenced syndromes like Alzheimer's and Huntington's, there are early manifestations (called *prodromal* features) that appear long before the clinical diagnosis and there is a characteristic developmental course after disease onset. So, even though neurological, psychiatric, and neurodevelopmental disorders have typically been studied separately, all three kinds of disorders should be explainable in a common theoretical framework. The application of such a framework will not only increase our scientific understanding of these disorders, but also improve prevention and treatment.

As we will see, there is a close, reciprocal relation between theories of normal function and explanations of disorders, and there is a continuing dialogue between discoveries in each domain. So, disorders have helped and continue to help us discover and analyze the components of the human mind in a way that studies of typical function sometimes cannot.

To understand these models of abnormal behavior, the reader needs to understand this dialogue. That is, the reader needs to understand the history and the original and later theoretical significance of each model. Issues over the interpretation of disorders lie at the heart of the field of cognitive neuroscience, both during its inception in the 19th century and today. The reader also needs to understand how these issues relate to broader issues in the philosophy of mind and the history of science, particularly biology. Consequently, the book begins with this broader context and then traces the history of continuing debates in cognitive neuroscience over the core issue of localization of function. As we will see, explanations of disorders often reveal core assumptions about how functions are localized and thus how the mind works. In fact, explaining all three kinds of disorders in a common framework is a very important test of the universality of our cognitive neuroscience models of normal and abnormal behavior and its development.

A final important point is that the seemingly sharp line drawn between normal and abnormal behavior starts to dissolve when we realize that the symptoms of many of these disorders lie on a continuum, with the cutoff for "disordered behavior" being somewhat arbitrary. So, it is inevitable that some individuals below the cutoff nonetheless have some of the defining symptoms. Moreover, rarer and seemingly pathognomonic symptoms can nonetheless be found in typical children at younger stages of development, and can be induced in typical adults by increasing their processing burden, revealing sometimes unexpected commonalities in the mechanisms underlying normal and abnormal behavior. The book will include relevant examples of seemingly pathognomonic symptoms that actually have analogues in typical development and in typical adults with reduced processing resources.

This book is divided into three main sections: (I) What Explanations Are Possible?, (II) What Are the Disorders?, and (III) What Becomes of the Self? The first section considers the history of neuroscience and the constraints that are placed on neuroscience explanations by the rest of science, including developmental science. It then presents cognitive neuroscience explanations of abnormal behavior, both classical and contemporary, and evaluates their scientific adequacy. The second section applies these models to disorders of all three types (neurological, psychiatric, and neurodevelopmental) in different domains of neuropsychological function: perception, attention, language, memory, action selection, emotion regulation, social perception and cognition, and global functioning. In each domain of function, we will briefly present contemporary theories of that particular normal function, including its development, and then evaluate how well those theories work to explain abnormal behavior in that domain. The final section examines the implications of the previous chapters for our conception of the self. To help the reader with technical terminology, this book includes a Glossary. The first time a technical term is used, it appears in bold print. There are also two Appendices to help the reader. Appendix A lists regions of the human neocortex by their names and Brodmann numbers and briefly describes their functions. Appendix B provides a list of online resources to help the reader learn more about neuroanatomy, functional neuroimaging, brain connectivity, neural network modeling, and genetics.

Acknowledgments

This book is dedicated to the memory of Guy Van Orden, PhD (10/2/1952–5/11/2012). Guy was my post doc (1985–1988) early in his illustrious career and had an enormous impact on my thinking about fundamental issues in neuropsychology. Guy earned his PhD in Cognitive Psychology from the University of California, San Diego, in 1984, a pivotal time and place in the history of psychology. Connectionism was being born through the efforts of Jay McClelland, Dave Rumelhart, and many collaborators, including Francis Crick, co-discoverer of the structure of DNA and a Nobel laureate. Guy absorbed this new approach to cognitive psychology and devoted his scientific career to exploring the implications of complexity science for psychology, in particular for the psychology of reading.

Guy and I had many discussions of how connectionist models and complex systems applied to dyslexia, both acquired and developmental. He slowly persuaded me that the localization of function paradigm in classical neuropsychology was fundamentally wrong. This was startling news for a clinical neuropsychologist in the mid-1980s!

The localization of function paradigm from 19th-century neurology had recently been revived by the new field of cognitive neuropsychology and was being applied to cases of acquired dyslexia. This research led to a very influential cognitive model of skilled single-word reading (i.e., the dual-route model, which had separate lexical and nonlexical routes for pronouncing a printed word). Guy was very critical of this model and the theoretical and empirical arguments that supported it. From a connectionist perspective, completely independent and separately localized routes or modules for different cognitive components of single-word reading did not make sense. In my lab, Guy began testing patients with Alzheimer's dementia on the reading paradigms used to diagnose different subtypes of acquired dyslexias predicted by dual-route theory. Surprisingly, many of these patients with diffuse neocortical damage showed error patterns similar to those found in acquired dyslexia subtypes. This pilot work and our many discussions led Guy to formulate a critique of double dissociation logic and we began working together on this topic. The result was a paper (Van Orden, Pennington, & Stone, 2001) that finally appeared in print 13 years later.

After working with Guy, my whole theoretical approach to neuropsychology and to psychology in general was transformed, and I slowly developed a new theoretical perspective, which is embodied in this book. Had it not been for Guy's influence, I would have gotten there a lot later, if at all.

This book has also benefited from the help of numerous collaborators and students. Anne B. Arnett, my last graduate student, did a superb job on the illustrations and end-of-chapter exercises. She and Robin Peterson carefully read earlier drafts, helping me to make the text clearer and more accurate.

Dorothy Bishop, Chris Filley, Michael Frank, Dan Leopold, Kateri McRae, Yuko Munakata, Randy O'Reilly, Jeremy Reynolds, Rob Roberts, Gerry Taylor, and Keith Owen Yeates read the near-final draft and made useful suggestions. My good friend (and exercise partner) Rich Mangen patiently listened to me expound on ideas in the book, and provided helpful comments on an earlier draft. Tejas Srinivas and Lisa Ankeny carefully proofread the page proofs.

My longtime administrative assistant, Suzanne Miller, provided invaluable help with this book, as she has with the three previous ones. I have *finally* learned to do most of my writing on a PC instead of by hand and to actually provide her with correct sources for the articles and books I cite in the text.

I also want to thank Seymour Weingarten and Rochelle Serwator at The Guilford Press for encouraging me to pursue this book and for all their help with my previous books. The whole production staff at Guilford has been very helpful.

Finally, my wife, Linda, has supported me throughout the writing of this book, as she has for my earlier three books. Our two grown children, Amy and Luke, have done so as well. During the writing of this book, I was also blessed with the arrival of my first grandchild, Della Dongching Lee Pennington (b. 12/15/2012), Luke and Lori's first child. "Dongching" is Mandarin for "light in the winter," and she is already a beacon of happiness for Linda and me.

Contents

PART I

WHAT EXPLANATIONS ARE POSSIBLE?

CHAPTER 1

Scientific Explanation

What does it mean to explain something? Basically, it means that we identify the cause of that thing in terms of relevant mechanisms. To elaborate this idea, let us consider the everyday example of a light switch (Rothman & Greenland, 1998, discussed in Rutter, 2006). If I flick the switch when the light is off, the light goes on. If I flick it when the light is on, the light goes off. This example corresponds pretty closely to our naive sense of what a single cause is, and also to how we test causality in science. By manipulating the hypothesized cause, we can either produce or eliminate the relevant outcome. A similar procedure is followed when testing new medical treatments and in brain stimulation studies.

Let's say the light doesn't come on when we flick the switch. Now there is a "disorder" that has eliminated (or, as we will say later, "subtracted") the function of the light. But what is the cause of this disorder? That is not so straightforward. If I replace the switch, will I cure the disorder? Possibly so, but possibly not. There could be lots of other things wrong instead, both things we can see and things we cannot. Maybe the lightbulb burned out, maybe a fuse has blown, maybe rodents chewed through the wires in the walls, maybe a tree fell on the power lines to the house, or maybe the power grid is down. This means that flicking the light switch is a necessary cause, but not a sufficient one; thus it is not actually a single cause of the lightbulb going off and on. Even in such a simple case as this, the apparent single cause is not actually single.

Let's carry this example a little further. The switch is a necessary but not sufficient cause of the state of the lightbulb (on vs. off), but can we set a boundary on the sufficient causes? We have already mentioned wiring and the power grid, but then the power grid depends on energy

3

generation, which usually depends on fossil fuels or renewable sources like wind and water. The energy in both of these sources depends on the sun, but the formation of our earth and sun depends on the history of the universe itself. Since the light switch and bulb are part of a system embedded in wider and wider systems, we really cannot set a boundary on sufficient causes. Moreover, these systems obey certain laws of physics, and designing the light switch, bulb, and all the rest depends on these laws. There are also levels of analysis in this example, ranging from the universe itself, to our particular planet and sun, to the power grid and its energy sources, down to the electrical system in our house, and eventually all the way down to the electrons that flow through the wires. So, the full answer to the question of what causes the light to come on is much more complicated than it first appears. What's important is that everything we know theoretically and empirically about these levels of analysis places very strict constraints on how the lightbulb and switch could work.

What we have learned from this example is that the mere observation of a functioning light, wherein we see that the sequence of "first, flick switch, then light turns on (or off)," can mislead us about the actual explanation of the phenomenon. Unfortunately, these naive conclusions abound in the history of science. The way things appear to happen has often misled us about actual causes, and the correct interpretation of observations has depended on theory. For example, the sun appears to rise in the morning and set at night, as if it were circling the earth (the geocentric hypothesis), and humans had no reason to doubt this conclusion until well into the 17th century. The truth, that the earth revolves around the sun (the heliocentric hypothesis), was not accepted until Galileo and others looked beyond the simplest, most apparent evidence, which was available in the most immediate system (not unlike the light switch), to test the alternative theory. Galileo's telescope allowed astronomers and citizens to consider evidence in a broader system. Thus, moving beyond the information gleaned from our casual observations (our phenomenology) depends on generating alternative explanations (hypotheses or theoretical models) and systematically testing them.

What happens to our explanations of phenomena when we move to living things and their organs? All that we have already said applies, but there are a few extra considerations. We can introduce a new kind of cause, functions that serve adaptive goals, as long as we locate these in the context of evolution. As Dobzhansky (1973) famously said, "nothing in biology makes sense except in the light of evolution." So, unlike the case with nonliving things, living things have functions and goals that explain their behavior, and this kind of teleological explanation is scientifically acceptable. Together, an organism's behavior can be explained by (1) distal goals that derive from its evolution (and from its development, in certain animals like humans with a long developmental period); and (2) proximal, mechanistic explanations based on the interactions of the organism's component parts (Goldsmith, 1991). The second, mechanistic explanation is similar to the light switch example. So, if we ask what causes vision in an animal, we can either frame the answer in terms of the eye and its connection to the brain (a proximal explanation in terms of the mechanism of vision), or in terms of why eyes and brains evolved to enable vision (a distal explanation in terms of evolved functions).

Neuroscience, and cognitive neuroscience within it, are interdisciplinary fields that share core assumptions with all of science and have similar criteria for what counts as an explanation for a phenomenon. These core assumptions are (1) **naturalism** or **materialism**, (2) **reductionism**, (3) **consilience**, (4) **empiricism**, and, increasingly, (5) **reconstructionism**. What does each of these core assumptions assert?

First, *naturalism* requires that any explanation be couched in terms of objects and forces of the natural, physical world. Thus, unlike in religion or mythology, supernatural beings or forces are excluded as possible explanations. This first tenet makes it clear why there has often been conflict between science and religion and why earlier scientists were sometimes literally risking their lives or their freedom (think of Giordano Bruno, who was burned at the stake partly for asserting there were multiple suns in the universe, or Galileo, who was forced to recant his heliocentric theory of the solar system) in doing their research. The same was true for early neuroscientists such as Thomas Willis (Zimmer, 2004), whose scientific theories challenged popular religious doctrine about the role of the soul in human behavior.

Reductionism requires that the explanation of a complex phenomenon, like the mind, lies in the interaction among simpler parts, like neurons. Rumelhart and McClelland and other connectionists (known as the Parallel Distributed Processing [PDP] Group; Rumelhart, McClelland, & the PDP Research Group, 1986) said that the key challenge for explaining cognition was how to "make a smart machine out of dumb parts," that is, neurons. Much of the history of neuroscience has been focused on reduction: discovering what the simpler parts of the brain are at various levels of analysis. So most neuroscience research begins with behavior and tries to reduce it to brain. This reduction is indicated in Figure 1.1 by the left arrow going down from Mind to Brain. In functional neuroimaging studies, this is called "forward inference." Every scientific discipline has elementary units (be they the elementary particles and forces of physics,

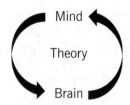

FIGURE 1.1. The ultimate goal of neuropsychology.

the elements in chemistry, or cells and genes in biology) whose interaction explains complex phenomena like rainbows, combustion, and life.

Consilience is a term used by E. O. Wilson (1998) to refer to what philosophers of science call the "network theory" of scientific truth. What this means is that any proposed scientific explanation must be consistent with everything else we already know across all of science. This is a very useful and demanding constraint on scientific explanations, one that can reject or at least seriously question some explanations at the outset. For instance, proposing that a dysfunctional grammar gene explains the lack of past-tense markers in members of the KE family (Gopnik & Crago, 1991) is inconsistent with how genes work to influence behavior (through many intervening levels of analysis) and how many human genes there are (about 25,000 for the entire body, which is not enough for a genetic phrenology). An innate, hardwired syntax module or face recognition module is inconsistent with what we know about brain development because synapses are mostly formed after birth and are "wired up" under the influence of activity and experience. So, what we know about the roles of genes and environments in shaping the developing nervous system imposes very important constraints on cognitive neuroscience explanations of abnormal behavior that are often overlooked. What we have learned about the plasticity of the human nervous system poses a similar constraint.

Empiricism requires that any scientific theory be testable and tested with actual experiments on entities in the natural world. Empiricism is what makes science progressive and allows debates between different theories to be settled, at least eventually. So, unlike debates in the popular media, everyone is not "entitled to their own opinion" in science. The opinions of scientists are subjected to rigorous scrutiny, both theoretical and empirical, before they can be accepted as valid. The goal of this scrutiny is to disconfirm or reject the theory being tested (Popper, 1959), not to confirm it. A theory that cannot be disconfirmed is accepted provisionally, meaning that it can always be disconfirmed by later tests.

Reconstructionism requires that we test a reductionistic explanation by seeing if it can reproduce the complex phenomenon it was supposed to explain, and this reproduction involves **emergent properties**, which are explained below. In Figure 1.1, the right arrow going up from Brain to Mind indicates reconstruction. Reconstruction is a newer requirement for scientific theories, especially in biology and the social sciences, because it requires computational models that were not feasible before the invention of modern computers. In functional neuroimaging studies, this reconstruction is called "reverse reference," explained below. Another way of explaining this tenet of a scientific explanation is to say that a mature scientific theory is mathematical. Increasingly, we hear about computational biology, and in neuroscience, computational models are crucial at several levels of analysis, from the actions of individual neurons to the interactions among brain regions.

Cells, organs, brains, societies, and economies are all examples of complex systems with *emergent properties* that derive from the interactions of their components. For example, the tertiary structure of a protein (the way the linear chain of its amino acids folds up) is an emergent property that is crucial for its function: how it can act either as a channel, a receptor, or a transporter of specific molecules. Many of the important functional properties of the nervous system emerge in development, so an important corollary of reconstructionism for neuroscience is that we cannot completely understand a brain function such as language or face perception without understanding its development.

Generally, a scientific investigation of a phenomenon begins with reduction, analogous to taking the light switch apart to examine its components, and eventually proceeds to reconstruction, once a fairly mature understanding of the phenomenon has been attained. Typically, different methods are used in these two phases of explanation, and the same is true in neuroscience. The last two centuries of neuroscience have focused mainly on reduction, but enough knowledge has accumulated that reconstruction has become possible and there is now a burgeoning field of systems neuroscience. The methods needed for these two phases of neuroscience are different, and the invention of new methods has greatly facilitated both phases of development in neuroscience. The reduction or analytic phase has relied on acquired and experimental lesions (what is lost when this part is removed?), behavioral dissociations and double dissociations, single-unit recordings (what does this particular neuron respond to?), and neuroimaging methods such as the subtraction method (i.e., neuroimaging studies that begin with behavioral contrasts in order to identify brain regions correlated with component processes of the behavior). The goal of these methods has been to isolate and localize component functions to discrete parts of the machine that is the brain. The reconstruction, or synthetic, phase relies on a number of different methods, all of which examine how the collective action of these individual parts gives rise to behavior. These methods include (1) neural network simulations of typical and atypical behavior, (2) analyses of brain structural and functional connectivity to identify neural systems, and (3) using multivariate methods to predict the behavioral state of the subject from the outputs of multiple single units or functional magnetic resonance imaging (fMRI) voxels as inputs (e.g., Poldrack, Halchenko, & Hanson, 2009), an example of what is called **reverse inference**. The first method is intrinsically developmental, whereas the latter two methods can be used to elucidate brain–behavior development.

It is hard to emphasize the importance of development enough because we cannot fully understand how the adult brain works without understanding how it developed. Any explanation of typical or atypical behavior that contradicts what we know about brain–behavior development is not tenable simply because it is impossible (it violates the consilience principle), unless that explanation can lead to a complete and consistent revision of our knowledge and theories of brain–behavior development. In this book, we will use these five principles to constrain explanations of different domains of brain function and the disorders that arise in those domains. A considerable amount of what will be presented in Part II on disorders demonstrates what has been learned from taking a reductionistic approach (the left arrow in Figure 1.1) to different domains of function. But we will also apply the constraints imposed on reductionistic explanations by the requirement for reconstruction (the right arrow in Figure 1.1). Part III will be mainly focused on reconstruction, particularly in the context of a neural explanation of self and consciousness.

CHAPTER 2

■■■■■■■■

Placing Neuroscience in the History of Science and Philosophy

The scientific study of neuroscience entailed taking a materialistic view of mind, in contrast to the dualist notion of mind's independence from body, a belief that went back to antiquity and was part of Christian doctrine. As will next be described, the debate over dualism paralleled earlier debates in the history of biology (Table 2.1). These debates bear on our main topic of explaining abnormal behavior because in each debate it became clear that the complex forms that were the topic of debate each required an explanation in terms of emergent properties. One of the main arguments of this book is that the explanation for abnormal behavior requires a similar kind of explanation: abnormal behavior is nearly always an emergent property of the interaction among components of a complex system, and not simply due to the absence of a single component.

As far back as Aristotle, there was controversy over how the form of an organism arose in development: Was it already preformed in the sperm or the egg (the **preformation theory**) or did it develop? Aristotle presciently argued for the latter position, which he called **epigenesis**, meaning literally that the organism's form arose "upon formation," and not before. But the preformationist doctrine, which made claims such as the existence of a small human inside the sperm or egg, persisted for many centuries. This hypothetical little person was called a "homunculus" and this kind of argument is still known as homuncular. The homunculus of preformationism had at least two fatal logical flaws. The first fatal flaw in preformationist arguments is that they do not explain what formed the homunculus in the first place. When one posits a prior and external cause for the form of an organism (i.e., the homunculus), the problem of explanation is only deferred. So that which is to be explained, the explanandum, is used as the explanation itself, resulting in circular reasoning. The second fatal flaw in the homunculus theory is that it predicted an endless regress of smaller and smaller homunculi since each homunculus had to contain not only its own form, but also the forms of all subsequent generations. Could there be an endless series of homunculi within homunculi, like Russian dolls? Would not a physical limit eventually be reached for the size of these ever smaller and smaller homunculi? Moreover, how could this theory explain why children were not identical copies of one parent or the other? Why were two parents needed at all? Another puzzle was how could new species arise. Only with the advent of the study of embryology and Darwin's theory of evolution in the 19th century was the preformationist theory finally rejected, at least in science.

Let's examine the second example in Table 2.1, the question of what causes life in an organism. The fact that organisms move of their own accord in a purposeful way and have other characteristics that distinguish them from nonliving things makes it tempting to infer that some special force underlies life, one that is unquestionably lost when the organism dies. This special force was termed the *élan vital* (vital or life force). So, once again the explanation of a mystery about living things was deferred to an external cause, which itself is not explained. The notion of the *élan vital* fell out of favor with the development of chemistry as a science and the subsequent discovery that living things were composed of chemicals (combination of elements) just as were nonliving things. The key difference was that the chemicals found in living things were usually much more complex compounds than the compounds found in nonliving things. So it now became feasible, at least in principle, to explain life in terms of the interactions of material things, without positing a special life force. The subsequent history of organic chemistry and biology has proven this to be the case. In that history, scientists have gone all the way

TABLE 2.1. Issues in the History of Biology

	External cause	Internal cause
Development	Preformation	Epigenesis
Life	*Élan vital* (life force)	Cell doctrine
Organs	Intelligent design	Natural selection
Mind	Dualism	Materialism

from synthesizing the organic molecules found in living things from simpler inorganic chemicals to recently constructing an artificial unicellular organism out of these same organic molecules. So, modern biology has proven that no vital force is need to account for living organisms, even though the idea of the *élan vital* is still embraced by some philosophers (e.g., Bergson, 1907).

The third example in Table 2.1 is the origin of living species themselves and their specialized organs. Darwin's theory of evolution by natural selection provided a mechanism whereby organs and species could arise without an external designer. His deeply counterintuitive theory was opposed during his time, and even today by those who maintain that such special structures as a human eye or an entire animal required an external designer. This latter position is called "intelligent design" or the "argument from design" (Dawkins, 1987). Once again, the explanation of a mystery invokes an external and nonmaterial cause, and so is not really an explanation at all. Where did the designer come from, who designed him or her, how is a nonmaterial being able to act on the material world, and so on? Again, the modern synthesis of Darwinian evolution and Mendel's genetics has tested and retested the adequacy of Darwin's theory for explaining the design of organs and organisms. For rapidly reproducing organisms, like bacteria and viruses, or rapidly reproducing cancer cells, we can observe evolution in the laboratory. We can even observe evolution in a patient's own body if he or she has cancer or a virus like HIV. In these latter cases, virtually every treatment can unfortunately lead to a new round of evolution of cancer cells or viruses so that they become resistant to that treatment. So, the patient is literally losing a race with evolution.

The final example in Table 2.1 is the central problem in neuroscience, the **mind–body problem**. What is the mind–body problem? Basically, it is the puzzle of how a physical body or, more specifically, a brain can have a mind with thoughts and feelings. Or to put it another way, how can consciousness arise from a physical system? In classical philosophy, the puzzle of *qualia* is closely related to the mind–body problem. *Qualia* (Latin for "qualities") are first-person, phenomenal experiences, such as our vivid experience of the redness of a rose, and thus are a part of a consciousness that itself needs to be explained. Such phenomenal experiences were a puzzle for classical philosophers because they seemed inconsistent with the materialistic requirement that the brain is a physical machine. No other machine they could think of, even an automaton, seemed likely to have qualia. Part of their conceptual problem was that they assumed that materialism entailed mechanism, and strict mechanism posed problems not only for how the mind worked but also for how life worked. As discussed in Chapter 1, living things are not just machines whose behavior is explained only by the proximal causes in their mechanism, they are also evolved organisms with adaptive functions (distal causes) based on their evolutionary history. Consciousness in humans and some other animals surely evolved, so there are both proximal and distal explanations for consciousness. When we discuss perception, we will return to the problem of qualia and review what has been learned about how the physical brain can simulate the external world.

One answer to the mind–body problem, and the qualia problem within it, is the dualistic answer. In its oldest form, the dualistic explanation simply denies that consciousness could arise from a physical system and posits instead that it is composed of a different substance. Dualism is an ancient idea in both Western and Eastern thought. For instance, Plato, in the 5th century B.C.E., held a dualist theory of mind, and Hindu thinkers around the same time proposed a similar theory. This explanation of the mind–body problem is called **substance dualism** and was elaborated by the philosopher Descartes. Many people in contemporary Western society are dualists and believe in what can be called "popular dualism." Popular dualism holds that the soul or mind survives the death of the body, and that therefore there can be ghosts or spirits. We can see the problem with dualism is similar to the problem posed by preformationism, vitalism, and intelligent design. In explaining a mystery, we invoke an external cause, which is itself an even greater mystery.

These four positions are all examples of the argument from incredulity (Churchland, 1995): "I cannot possibly understand how this phenomenon could arise from material causes, so there must be some radically different explanation." We can see why the argument from incredulity just generates greater incredulity because it posits a mysterious force that cannot be observed or tested.

Moreover, the split between mind and body is not as great as it first appears, or as appears to a philosopher who is thinking in abstract sentences. Much of our mental experience is about *bodily* states, whether internal ones (interoceptive states, like hunger, thirst, sexual desire, the need to eliminate, and so on), external or exteroceptive perceptual experiences (like vision, hearing, touch, smell, and taste), or somatosensory states of the body in action (proprioceptive states). In addition, our seemingly abstract concepts are themselves rooted in bodily experience (embodied cognition), as explained by Lakoff (1987) and Johnson (1990). Given the close connections between our bodies and our mental states, how could a disembodied mind even have a mental life? As tough as the mind–body problem is, the "mind-without-body problem" is even tougher.

Progress is actually being made on the mind–body problem, just as it has already been made on the three other problems of biology in Table 2.1, which have now been essentially solved. If we divide the mind–body problem into a continuum of subproblems, we can see that science has made considerable progress in solving several of them. This continuum of subproblems begins with the life–matter and the matter–computation problems, which have been solved. We know how material biological systems support life, and we have created silicon-based computers and robots that can perform computations. The next subproblem, the brain–behavior problem—How does a material brain perform the computations that cause behavior?—is the main focus of neuroscience, and considerable progress has been made in solving it. The neural circuits underlying many behaviors have been elucidated and simulated, as we will see in subsequent chapters in this book. The last subproblem—Why and how does this neuronal computer, our brain, gives rise to consciousness?—is referred to by Chalmers (1998) as the "hard problem" of consciousness, but having solved or nearly solved the previous subproblems has certainly brought us closer to solving the *hard problem*.

The mind–body problem is also a developmental problem, and subsequent chapters of this book consider what we have learned about the development of the various neural circuits that support behavior. One can more specifically ask about the development of human consciousness: when and how does consciousness arise in human infants and young children? To answer that question, we must first distinguish different kinds of consciousness: being awake, having interoceptive experiences, having exteroceptive qualia, having self-awareness, having retrospective experience (episodic memory), prospective experience, and interpersonal experience. Neonates have some of these, but not all of them (Koch, 2009; Kostovic & Judas, 2010). Similarly, the mind–body problem is an evolutionary and comparative problem: which neural circuits that support behavior are common across different species? With respect to consciousness in particular, one can ask how many of the kinds of consciousness just listed are present in various animal species, and how did the neural mechanisms for each one evolve?

Similar to my argument above, Prinz (2005) shows that four important components of the consciousness problem are yielding to empirical analysis. He calls these four (1) the "what" problem (Of which states are we conscious and which not?), (2) the "where" problem (What parts of the brain are necessary for consciousness?), (3) the "how" problem (How do certain mental states become conscious?), and (4) the "who" problem (Who has consciousness?)—similar to the developmental and comparative issues just discussed. With regard to the "what" problem, cognitive neuroscience has clearly demonstrated that many cognitive operations occur outside of conscious awareness, from the extraction of low-level sensory features in the retina and primary visual cortex (V1) and other sensory systems, to unconscious emotional reactions to certain subliminal stimuli, to the vestibular ocular reflex, which tells us to disregard changes in the perceived world generated by our own movements. Prinz argues that we are mainly conscious of the products of intermediate-level perceptual processes in the neocortex, but only when these are attended to. So attention is part of the answer to the "how" problem, and we will see later that without attention, major parts of the present world will be neglected by both typical individuals and patients with certain kinds of lesions.

With regard to the "where" problem, recent research supports the view that consciousness is not localized, but instead an emergent property of the whole brain and nervous system. We also know about different states of consciousness, from brain death to normal waking consciousness (see Figure 2.1), and we can distinguish these states by their patterns of electroencephalographic (EEG) or fMRI activity in the neocortex. In this figure based on Bernat, 2009, and Sanders, 2012, various states of consciousness are distinguished by observable criteria. These states can be more precisely measured with EEG and fMRI. EEG exhibits different wave patterns (based on frequency) in different states of consciousness. So, gamma waves (30–100 Hz) are one EEG signature of consciousness; later research has examined gamma synchrony across cortical areas as an index of the activity necessary for an integrated conscious experience (Singer & Gray, 1995). In contrast, deep, nondreaming sleep is characterized by slow rhythmic delta waves (<4 Hz). As will be discussed in Chapter 13, the activity of the so-called **default mode network** (**DMN**; see Plate 13.1) indexes conscious activity at rest when an individual is thinking by him- or herself. Medial cortical brain structures such as the **precuneus** are part of the DMN and have the highest level of cerebral blood flow when a person is awake and aware. So DMN activity could provide an even more precise objective measure of consciousness. Thus, the cortex appears to be at least necessary for conscious awareness and hence part of the answer to the "where" problem.

As discussed in Churchland (Churchland, 2013 #5738), when we are conscious, the central thalamus activates every portion of the neocortex

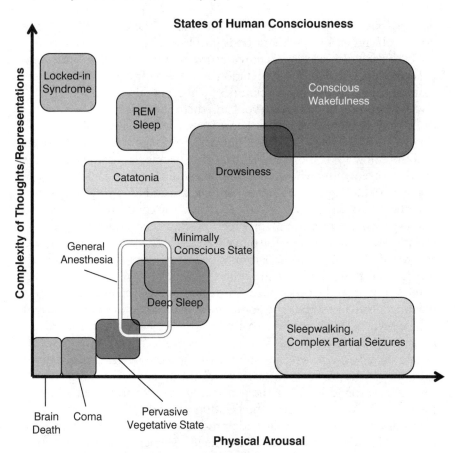

FIGURE 2.1. Normal and abnormal states of consciousness. Based on Bernat (2009) and Sanders (2012).

permitting the interactions among various parts of the neocortex that mediate conscious experience. These interactions are facilitated by the "small world" connectivity pattern in the brain in which local clusters are connected with each other through a few hubs or nodes. The inputs from the central thalamus and the small world connectivity pattern are consistent with the *global workspace theory* of consciousness (Baars, 1989).

The really hard part of the mind–body problem is the other "how" problem: how certain physical states in the body are possibly experienced by the mind (Chalmers, 1998). As previously discussed, this hard problem of consciousness is not as hard as its alternative, the experience-without-body problem, or mind-without-body problem. These four questions form the basis for a new science of consciousness within cognitive neuroscience (Baars & Gage, 2010); the expectation among cognitive neuroscientists is that the hard problem of consciousness will eventually be solved.

Besides the mind–body problem, there are other perennial issues in the philosophy of mind that neuroscience will likely eventually solve. These issues include the origin of human knowledge (the epistemological problem), how we come to know that other people have minds (the other minds problem), and whether we have free will. The two classical answers to the epistemological problem are **empiricism** and **idealism**. Very simply put, these two classical answers hold that knowledge either results from our experience (empiricism) or precedes experience (idealism). Consequently, idealism must posit a source for ideas outside of experience, such as a world of ideal forms in Platonism or innate rational structures in the mind, as proposed by Kant and other philosophers. We can see that this issue is similar to the other puzzles in Table 2.1, as well as to the nature–nurture debate in psychology. Sometimes, the resolution to an intractable debate such as this is to show that *both* sides are wrong. For the nature–nurture debate, Oyama (1985) persuasively argued that both sides of the debate shared an erroneous premise, that the form of the organism must exist outside the processes through which the organism develops, and that this form is found in either the genome (nature) or in the environment (nurture). As we said earlier, the position supported by modern biology is that form arises in an epigenetic process in which there is a constant interplay between genes and environment. Similarly, Piaget's constructivist (and developmental) answer to the epistemological problem is that knowledge develops out of the interplay between innate constraints in the human nervous system and environmental inputs.

The other minds problem is the question of how we know that other people have minds and how we have knowledge of what is in their minds. The other minds problem lies at the heart of the study of social cognition, and we will see that cognitive neuroscience is beginning to provide answers to this problem. To appreciate the other minds problem, let us return to Prinz's (2005) "who" problem. We readily make the inference that other adult humans are conscious when they are awake, acting purposefully, and especially when they are interacting with us. What the other minds problem highlights is that we do not have direct, first-person experience of another person's consciousness, so our attribution of consciousness to them must be just that—an attribution or inference. To highlight this fact, philosophers introduced the "zombie" problem. Maybe other people we think are conscious could really be zombies (or robots) who are programmed to provide an extremely convincing simulation of consciousness. How do we know for sure that we are not talking to a zombie instead of a real human being? Even though we cannot refute the zombie hypothesis directly, we can use the consilience principle to reject it. Would it make sense for evolution to endow just one human being with consciousness and have all the others be zombies? Not when you consider all the other converging biological evidence that other humans are constructed the same way I am.

The interesting aspect of the other minds problem is the question of how far consilience will take us when we start to consider whether very young or atypical human beings are conscious and which types of consciousness are found in various nonhuman animal species. Which types of consciousness are present in the fetus (Koch, 2009; Kostovic & Judas, 2010)? The neonate? An anencephalic child (Merker, 2007; Shewmon, Holmes, & Byrne, 1999)? A monkey? A rat? A snake? A cricket? In each of these cases, the organism in question may behave in ways that elicit our attribution of consciousness, but the attribution may be mistaken (i.e., a case of anthropomorphizing).

Finally, we come to the problem of free will versus determinism. It is a staple of folk psychology and common law that human adults possess free will—that we are rational agents who consciously decide which actions to perform and which not to perform. But a scientific explanation of human behavior only admits of the proximal and distal causes discussed in Chapter 1. Such an explanation can, and probably must, include consciousness, but it does not include the freedom to suddenly do something that nothing in our past could have predicted (as many lay people likely believe). Wegner (2002) has provided considerable evidence that our experience of conscious will is an *inference* that we make, not a *direct experience* of our will making things happen in the world through the actions of our bodies. The telling evidence is that we can both attribute will when there is none and deny will when it is present (e.g., when using a Ouija board). The cognitive neuroscience of action selection and the perception of intentionality are also pertinent to this problem, as are disorders in which the experience of will is dissociated from an agent's purposeful actions. For instance, in the **alien-hand syndrome** (or even in **overflow movements** in typical development), the individual makes purposeful movements that are not perceived as willed. Similarly, in schizophrenia, the origins of the patient's own thoughts are attributed to an external source. All of these specific examples point to the conclusion that our experience of free will is a construction or inference that can go awry. Nonetheless, off-line planning and instruction can change our later actions and free us from the press of immediate circumstances. Human evolution and culture have led to this limited kind of free will. Still, even with training, our actions are traceable to the planning and instruction that precede them.

CHAPTER SUMMARY

In this chapter, we have considered three core problems in the history of biology that relate to neuroscience, namely the problems of the origins of living things, their development, and their evolution. In each case, science has been able to provide a naturalistic explanation of the phenomenon in question without resorting to forces or forms outside of the phenomenon itself. These explanations all demonstrate how more complex forms (emergent properties) can arise out of the interactions among simpler parts. Now the mystery of the most puzzling phenomenon of all, human and animal consciousness, is yielding to a similar approach. Similarly, other perennial puzzles in the philosophy of mind, namely the epistemological, other minds, and free will problems, are being illuminated by discoveries in cognitive neuroscience. Again the solution to these puzzles lies in emergent properties of a complex, natural system, and does not require some force or form outside of the phenomenon itself. However, materialism and naturalism should be regarded only as the starting assumptions of scientific explanations, not as dogmas. Just as has occurred in modern physics, in which our conceptions of the core entities of matter and energy have changed considerably since the beginning of the 20th century because of new discoveries, we should be open to discoveries that challenge core assumptions in current neuroscience. Such discoveries have already occurred and will undoubtedly continue.

EXERCISES

1. The Cambridge Declaration on Consciousness (*http://fcmconference.org/img/ CambridgeDeclarationOnConsciousness.pdf*), signed by a group of scientists at the Francis Crick Memorial Conference on Consciousness in Human and Non-Human Animals in July 2012, states that nonhuman animals do experience consciousness. This conclusion is based on the observation of animals' intentional behaviors, as well as indications of human-like brain substrates. They declare, "the absence of a neocortex does not appear to preclude an organism from experiencing affective states." Do you agree? What else,

beyond "affective states," is important in consciousness? How far down the animal kingdom chain would you find consciousness? Would you include birds? Fish? Beetles? Larvae? Have this debate with someone you know and along the way decide how you define consciousness and how that affects your position on these issues.

2. Search for "alien-hand syndrome" on YouTube and view some of the videos posted there. How is the mind–body problem complicated by this disorder?

CHAPTER 3

▪▪▪▪▪▪▪▪

History of the Localization of Function Debate

An act of speech is a march of events, where one changing condition passes insensibly into another. When speech is defective, this easy motion or transition is impeded; one state cannot flow into another. . . . So, when a break occurs in the functional chain, orderly speech becomes impossible, because the basic physiological processes which subserve it have been disturbed. The site of such a breach of continuity is not a "centre for speech," but solely a place where it can be interrupted or changed.

—HEAD (1926, p. 474)

Localized lesions produce symptoms which vary with the area involved, but the character of these symptoms is such as to preclude anatomical correlations significant for the problem of brain mechanisms. Localization as an explanatory principle can progress in only one way; by the demonstration of correspondences between ever more restricted anatomical divisions and smaller units of behavior until some ultimate anatomical and behavioristic elements are reached-the old notion of elementary ideas located in single cells in the brain.

—LASHLEY (1929, p. 162)

The goal of this chapter is to help the reader understand a key concept in neuroscience, namely, *localization of function*, by examining how this concept has evolved in the history of the field. This concept is pertinent to explaining abnormal behavior because loss of a localized function (called the *subtraction model*—see also Chapter 4, which reviews different models for explaining abnormal behavior) has been the dominant model in cognitive neuroscience for much of its history. A key theme of this book is that the appealingly simple subtraction model is too simple for explaining many abnormal behaviors, so it is very important for students of abnormal behavior to understand the shortcomings of this simple model. Just as normal functions at different levels of analysis are emergent properties of the interaction of multiple components of a complex system (as was explained in Chapters 1 and 2), so too is abnormal function.

Like foundational concepts in other fields, such as the concept of the *gene* in biology or *energy* in physics, the concept of localization of function has been subject to intense debate and continuing revision as the field has advanced. As the opening quotes make clear, reservations about localization of function have been trenchantly and repeatedly expressed in the history of neuroscience. Some early neuroscientists focused their attention on specialized centers for different brain functions, but others emphasized the connections between such centers (i.e., neural circuits), as the opening quotes by Head and Lashley make clear. But these reservations have often been forgotten by later generations of neuroscientists, who fall into the same conceptual errors that were criticized in the past. So it is important to understand both the history of this debate as well as how it is playing out today. There are three main parts of this chapter: (1) an overview of the history of the localization debate, (2) a more detailed discussion of the latest round in that debate, which has focused on a method called **double dissociation**, and (3) the recent discovery of various structural and functional networks in the brain and their role in abnormal behaviors. As we will see, arguments about the validity of the double dissociation method reprise some of the issues that arose earlier in debates over localization of function, and network models are finally resolving this debate by concretely demonstrating how centers and connections work together in the real brain.

Before starting on the first part of this chapter, on the history of the localization debate, a few clarifying points are important to bear in mind. First, location in the brain *does* matter. No one, not even Karl Lashley, claimed the brain is completely equipotential. In fact, the extreme position of **equipotentiality** is just as absurd as the opposite extreme position, which has come to be called the **grandmother cell hypothesis**, the idea that only a single neuron is dedicated to the representation of a single idea, such as the representation of an individual's grandmother. As we will see in Part II, brain structures that are located close together often have a family resemblance in their functions, simply because they share connections with each other. A pressing design constraint on the evolution of the brain is the need to make connections as short as possible. Neural wiring is expensive, just as it is in an artificial computer; the brain has evolved such that multiple "wires" work together to perform a variety of functions, rather than a single "wire" (neuron) corresponding to a single function. Thus, at a basic level, location is a rough but useful guide to what a structure might be doing.

Second, as discussed in Chapter 1, the full explanation of any function or dysfunction cannot be reduced to a single localized cause, as illustrated by the example of a light switch. A single cause (e.g., a localized lesion) may be sufficient to eliminate a brain function, but that cannot mean that the brain location is both necessary *and* sufficient for that function. Any function depends on a series of embedded physical systems, as we saw in the example of the light switch. A brain location is embedded in a brain, which is embedded in a body, which is embedded in a physical and social context, and so on.

Third, an apparent localization of function does not automatically entail an *innate* localization or lack of plasticity for that function. Such an apparent localization of function just means that *in the course of development* a brain structure has become specialized for that function. It is possible that other brain areas could have developed that brain function had there been different inputs during the developmental process. Also, for some functions, localization changes with development, as we will discuss in later chapters. So, it is an empirical question as to how innate or plastic different brain functions are. From what we already know, there is not a "one size fits all" answer to these questions for the whole of the human nervous system. Some functions are undoubtedly innate, such as breathing, sucking, an aversive reaction to a bitter taste, and some basic aspects of homeostatic regulation. Their innateness (i.e., presence from birth) does not mean they might not be plastic postnatally and certainly doesn't mean we therefore know how they developed prenatally. The degree of innateness of various functions is related to the evolutionary history of different parts of the brain. A guiding but hardly infallible principle is that the older the brain structure, the more innate its function is. For instance, the hypothalamus, brainstem, and the peripheral autonomic nervous system, which are all involved in homeostatic regulation, are evolutionarily ancient parts of the nervous system, and many of their functions are innate, such as the control of breathing, hunger, thirst, and temperature. Nonetheless, both the fetus (through prenatal programming) and later the infant learn different settings for these homeostatic functions based on the environment they encounter (Agin, 2010). On the other hand, if one of these ancient brain structures is absent or damaged, its function is usually lost, sometimes with fatal consequences. A different structure generally cannot take on that particular function. By contrast, the neocortex is a newer part of the brain evolutionarily, and it exhibits less functional commitment at birth and more plasticity than the structures just discussed. The intense debates in the field of neuropsychology have been mainly concerned with neocortical functions. For instance, is there an innate face module or language module? As will be seen in later chapters, the current state of the evidence does not support the existence of innate neocortical modules for these functions. Nonetheless, neocortical plasticity, while considerable, has important limits, and we will discuss those in Part II as we discuss different domains of function. With these three important points in mind, let us turn to the history of the localization debate in neuroscience.

RECURRING LOCALIZATION DEBATES

Shallice (1988) and others have noted that controversies over localization of function in neuropsychology have a "remarkable dialectical quality" (p. 6). In a dialectic, a theoretical position engenders an opposite position, and the clash of opposites leads to a new theoretical position, which again engenders its opposite, and so on, leading hopefully to increasingly adequate theories. Kuhn (1962) embraced a dialectical view of the evolution of scientific theories, and made the important point that competing theoretical paradigms can be so solipsistic that they often talk right past each other. This phenomenon can definitely be found in the continuing controversy about localization of function. In each round of the debate over localization of function, a localizationist claim has quickly given rise to an opposite, antilocalizationist claim and then a new synthesis (see Table 3.1). But the new synthesis never adequately addresses holistic reservations about localized functions, and so the debate recurs.

Round 1: Equipotentiality versus Phrenology

Although the notion that the brain is the organ of thought dates to antiquity, Franz Joseph Gall (1768–1828) is the first modern localizationist in the sense of both hypothesizing that different faculties have different brain regions devoted to them, and crucially, in using an empirical method to test these localizations (Gall & Spurzheim, 1809). Moreover, instead of using introspective philosophical analysis to decide what the faculties were, Gall derived his list of fundamental faculties from empirical observations of individual, gender, and species differences. Thus, besides being the first modern localizationist, Gall was also the first differential and comparative psychologist. Like Gardner's (1983) theory of multiple intelligences, Gall's faculty theory placed special weight on evidence from

TABLE 3.1. The Recurring Localization Debate

	Holistic		Localizationist	Outcome
Round 1: 1810–42	Marie Jean Pierre Flourens: Equipotentiality	vs. vs.	Franz Joseph Gall: Localized centers	Equipotentiality is supported.
Round 2: 1861	Flourens: Equipotentiality	vs. vs.	Pierre Paul Broca: Localized centers	There is a brain center for speech, so equipotentiality is rejected.
Round 3: 1874	Carl Wernicke: Multiple language centers	vs. vs.	Broca: Single language center	There are at least *two* language centers and a connection between them.
Round 4a: 1881–1920	Sigmund Freud, Pierre Marie, James Hughlings Jackson, Henry Head: Critics of localization	vs.	Wernicke and Ludwig Lichtheim: Diagram makers	The lesion that impairs a function does not necessarily tell you the location of that function. Pure cases may be a tautology.
Round 4b: 1929	Karl Lashley: Mass action	vs.	Wernicke and Lichtheim: Diagram makers	Reflex arcs and memories are not localized.
Round 5: 1960s– present	Connectionists: Distributed processing	vs.	Modern cognitive neuropsychologists: Double dissociation	Double dissociations do not necessarily reveal independent functions.

extreme individual differences observed in geniuses and savants. Despite the humorous mention usually given to Gall and his theory of phrenology in psychology textbooks, Gall was a serious scientist who originated ideas that are still influential today. Young (1970) makes this point in his careful analysis of the evolution of ideas about localization of function in the last century.

Fodor's (1983) influential book *The Modularity of Mind* takes its central thesis (i.e., there are localized faculties in the human brain, which Fodor terms "modules") from Gall, which is a remarkable example of how rejected ideas in neuroscience recur in later eras. In Fodor (1983), a cognitive module has these defining features: (1) it performs a specialized, evolved cognitive computation, such as speech or face perception; (2) it is localized in the neocortex; (3) it is innate (present from birth); and (4) it is informationally encapsulated, meaning that its dedicated computation is obligatory (e.g., we are unable to "turn off" perceiving speech or faces) and unaffected by neural computations occurring elsewhere (e.g., changes in attention). Fodor distinguished what he called "vertical" faculties, which are specialized for one particular domain of information, like speech or faces, from "horizontal" faculties, which operate across different domains of information, as attention or memory does. In Fodor's (1983) theory, only vertical faculties could be modular, whereas horizontal faculties could not. He went on to speculate that because horizontal faculties depend on distributed processing in the brain, we would forever lack a neuropsychology of such faculties, and hence a neuropsychology of thinking (since much of our thinking relies on attention and various kinds of memory).

Fodor's (1983) book was enormously influential in the new field of cognitive neuroscience, and many researchers accepted his arguments about the existence of cognitive modules and set out to find where they were in the brain. Modules were also very appealing on evolutionary grounds. The human brain had evolved to perform certain functions that were adaptive in the extended kinship groups of hunter-gatherers, and so it seemed plausible that certain human functions, like face perception, theory of mind, and aspects of language, such as phonology and syntax, could be examples of evolved innate cognitive modules. As we will see in later chapters, much of Fodor's modularity theory has been disproven by subsequent discoveries in neuroscience, and his prediction about the impossibility of a neuropsychology of horizontal faculties has been proven wrong. We have learned a considerable amount about the neuropsychology of horizontal faculties such as attention and various kinds of memory. Further, the vertical faculties hypothesized by Fodor have not turned out to be modular. What is important here is that Fodor (1983) based his modularity theory on the earlier and even more modular theory of brain functions developed by Gall and Spurzheim, to which we return.

Gall's thinking can be summarized as four core assumptions about localization of function:

1. Mental functions can be divided into innate, independent, domain-specific faculties. Some are common across species; others are unique to the human species. Although all faculties are species-typical, there are nonetheless individual differences within a species in how well developed a given faculty is.
2. Which faculties are independent and fundamental is determined by contrasting dissociations (implicitly, double dissociations)

within and between individuals, especially between individuals with extreme individual differences. Unlike later localizationists, however, Gall was extremely skeptical about what could be learned from lesions.

3. There is one-to-one mapping between brain structures and faculties.

4. There is also one-to-one mapping between the brain structures serving faculties and the shape of the skull.

Of these four assumptions, the last was the most contentious and the most quickly refuted. The first three assumptions, on the other hand, have persisted in neuropsychology and were embraced in Fodor's (1983) modularity theory. The third assumption, although contradicted by empirical findings of multiple centers for complex functions, is an extreme form of what is called the **transparency assumption**, which holds that there is a simple, clear mapping between brain and behavior. A related assumption is the subtraction assumption, which holds that a single function can be clearly subtracted from the brain, leaving all other functions undisturbed (these two assumptions define the popular **subtraction model** for explaining abnormal behavior, which is discussed further in Chapter 4). As we will see later, these two assumptions are also critical for both the double dissociation method and for the subtraction method in functional neuroimaging.

Other problems with Gall's research program were that it relied on correlations, rather than experiments, and that in practice, Gall and his followers showed a strong confirmation bias (Young, 1970). Of course, the latter two problems are still with us.

Gall's ideas were strongly opposed by other brain researchers of the time, who believed the cortex was equipotential. Chief among these was Flourens, who was one of the founders of experimental physiology. His lesion experiments on pigeons did not support localized functions in the cortex. He also opposed Gall's theories because he believed in Cartesian dualism and the unity of the soul or mind. Any division of the functions of the mind was, for him, equivalent to denying the existence of the soul. Other early physiologists, like Magendie and Muller, acknowledged the material basis of behavior. But like Flourens, they rejected both the localization of functions in the cortex, as well as any role for the cortex in the direct initiation of muscular movements (thus preserving a less extreme form of dualism). At the same time, these early physiologists viewed Magendie's discovery of localized sensory and motor roots in the spinal cord as fundamental for an understanding of nervous system function.

Notice that their views contained an apparent schism between a holistic view of the cortex and a reductionist view of the spinal cord. In sum, in the first round of the localization debate, holists prevailed over the phrenologists.

Round 2: Equipotentiality versus Cortical Centers

Flourens's equipotential view on the function of the cortex was contradicted by Broca's discovery of a left-hemisphere center for speech, and by later discoveries by Wernicke, Fritsch and Hitzig, and Ferrier. Broca described the first clinical localizations of function in the neocortex. Broca's (1861) report on the patient Tan who had a localized lesion in the left inferior frontal lobe (now Broca's area), and whose speech was markedly reduced, convinced neurologists of the time that there were localized functions in the cortex, as the phrenologists had claimed. Later experimental research convincingly demonstrated that the cortex was *not* equipotential. Fritsch and Hitzig (1870) demonstrated the first, widely accepted, experimental localization of function in the cortex. They stimulated the cortex of dogs electrically, finding areas that led to motor movements when stimulated. Ferrier (1886) extended this work to monkeys and other animals, showing that the concept of a motor cortex was a general mammalian feature, and he also demonstrated the localization of somatosensory cortex. Young (1970) argued that Ferrier's work extended the sensory–motor physiology Magendie found in the spine to the whole nervous system, so that one could think of its functions in terms of reflex arcs or associations between sensory inputs and motor outputs. In other words, the reductionism that Magendie resisted for cortex was implemented by Ferrier. To Young (1970), Gall's and Ferrier's theories had complementary strengths and weaknesses. Gall had an interesting, biologically plausible theory of functions but did not constrain it with any direct physiological knowledge. Ferrier, on the other hand, relied only on direct brain experiments but reduced all behavior to sensation and motion, enshrining associationist psychology in the brain.

Round 3: Single versus Multiple Language Centers

Although Broca's (1861) discovery of a localized center for speech appeared to confirm the phrenologists' theory that there were *single* cortical centers for various complex functions, the idea of single centers, at least for language, was quickly rejected. Carl Wernicke (1874) discovered a second language center in the posterior left hemisphere, lesions to which produced a different symptom profile from that found in Broca's patient Tan. The existence of *two* language centers prompted the question of how they worked together. Wernicke answered this question by proposing a simple anatomical and functional model in which Broca's area and Wernicke's areas were connected by a white matter tract called the **arcuate fasciculus**. This connection between the two language centers explained how it was possible to repeat speech that had been heard. (See Chapter 8 for a more detailed discussion of the discoveries of Broca and Wernicke.)

Round 4a: The Diagram Makers and Their Critics

The next round of the localization debate occurred in late-nineteenth-century aphasiology. Case studies by Broca, Wernicke, and others led to the creation of models consisting of centers and routes to explain and predict different subtypes of aphasia. These models are like the "box-and-arrow" models of the 20th-century information-processing theorists. In such a box-and-arrow model, the boxes represent stages of information processing and the arrows represent the flow of information from lower to higher stages of information processing. Two important assumptions of such box-and-arrow models are that information processing is unidirectional and serial. As we will see in the next chapter, there is now considerable evidence that information processing in the brain is, instead, bidirectional and parallel. Lichtheim's (1885) classic paper provided an early box-and-arrow model with three centers (boxes) and five pathways (arrows; see Figure 8.1).

In this paper, he also introduced the important distinction between pure and mixed cases. A pure case was one in which a single box or arrow was damaged, thus cleanly subtracting that function or connection and leaving the patient with a set of remaining functions that transparently reflected the remaining intact components. So the notion of a pure case depends on both the subtraction and transparency assumptions discussed earlier.

Lichtheim and other neurologists like Wernicke, who proposed such models, were pejoratively described as "diagram makers" by their critics. These critics included Marie (1906a), Freud (1891), Hughlings Jackson (1931), and Head (1926). Their criticisms put an end to this approach to aphasia, effectively ending the classical period of neuropsychology. These critics noted several problems: (1) the precise localizations posited by the diagram makers' theories did not always prove reliable in subsequent observations; (2) their theoretical concepts were not adequate to explain all the symptoms of aphasia (e.g., agrammatism); and (3) the behavioral documentation of their cases was weak and unsystematic. Repeatedly, in his famous paper, Lichtheim (1885) had to apologize that no data on this or that language function were collected from a given case that provided a critical test of his theory.

Perhaps the most telling criticism of the diagram makers was that of Head (1926), who emphasized that few cases were as pure as the theorists supposed: "As each case arose, it was lopped and trimmed to correspond with a lesion of some cortical center or hypothetical path" (p. 56). Essentially, theory adjudicated pure versus impure cases. Most important, Head questioned the independence assumption: "but most of them fell into the subtle error of assuming that the elements reached by analysis could be treated as independent entities, which had entered into combination" (p. 66). Head also critiqued the transparency and locality assumptions:

> Local destruction of the tissues of the brain prevents the normal fulfillment of some specific form of behavior, and the reaction which follows expresses the response of the organism as a whole to the new situation. No function, somatic or physical, is a mosaic of elementary processes which become manifest when it is disturbed in consequence of a cerebral lesion. (Head, 1926, p. 548)

Round 4b: Mass Action versus Diagram Makers

Early in the 20th century, Karl Lashley contributed empirical results that strongly questioned two localizations of function, the reflex arc and a discrete location for a given memory. Ferrier's associationist assumption of localized cortical reflex arcs was falsified by Lashley (1929, 1950). Lashley used lesions to disconnect sensory from motor cortex in experimental animals but found no loss of the ability to learn a new conditioned response. He said, "Such arcs are either diffused through all parts of the cortex, pass by relay through lower centers, or do not exist" (Lashley, 1950, p. 461). Lashley also conducted lesion experiments to test whether new memories were localized and found they were stored in a distributed rather than localized fashion. Lashley proposed that the "engram of a new association, far from consisting of a single bond or neuron connection, is probably a reorganization of a vast system of associations involving the interrelations of hundreds of thousands or millions of neurons" (1950, p. 475). To account for his results from these lesion experiments, Lashley proposed the principle of **mass action**. This principle holds that the effect of a lesion on a function like a memory or a reflex depends not on its location but on the size of the lesion: bigger lesions produced more loss of function.

Summary of Rounds 1–4

These rounds of the localization debate confronted a variety of embedded issues. Flourens's opposition to Gall was mainly a defense of dualism, whereas Wernicke's critique of Broca's localization hypothesis focused on the issue of single versus multiple centers (with connections between them). In the early 20th century, several proponents of holism, including Head (1926), Goldstein (1948), and Lashley (1950), criticized the diagram makers' models of spoken and written language that had evolved in the latter part of the 19th century because these models lacked explanatory adequacy and the observations supporting them were often unreliable.

Round 5: The Double Dissociation Debate

We now arrive at Round 5 (see Table 3.1) in the localization debate, which is still going on. A key issue in this round of the debate is the significance of double dissociations. In modern cognitive neuroscience, localizationists have developed and utilized much more powerful experimental methods to identify independent components of mind. These methods include cognitive experiments and neuroimaging studies. One key method in these cognitive experiments has been to test for double dissociations. This test involves finding two contrasting single dissociations in two patient groups with different localized lesions, thus producing a crossover interaction. Because there are two opposite single dissociations, the entire pattern of results is called a "double dissociation." So in a double dissociation, Group 1 is impaired on Task A but not on Task B, whereas Group 2 shows the opposite profile (see Figure 3.1). When this pattern of results is found, the localizationist inference is that Task 1 and Task 2 require qualitatively different functions served by independent modules with separate brain mechanisms. (See Van Orden et al., 2001, for a fuller discussion of these issues.)

A simple example can illustrate what a double dissociation is, as well as some of the subtleties involved in interpreting what it means. Consider a group (1) with congenital (or acquired) peripheral blindness (because of selective damage to the eyes) and a second group (2) with congenital (or acquired) peripheral deafness (because of selective damage to the ears). Group 1 is selectively impaired in the function of vision (A) but has intact hearing, whereas Group 2 is selectively impaired in the function of hearing (B) but has intact vision. This pattern of results constitutes a classic double dissociation as seen in Figure 3.1 and seemingly warrants the straightforward interpretation that the eyes are specialized for peripheral vision and the ears are specialized for peripheral hearing. The subtleties arise when one starts thinking about *central* vision and hearing in these two groups. Now, because of brain plasticity, things are not as clearcut. As discussed in Chapter 5, individuals with blindness or deafness remap the preserved sensory input (hearing or vision, respectively) onto the primary sensory cortex (visual or auditory, respectively) that is no longer receiving peripheral input. So, sensation and perception in the preserved sensory modality are *enhanced above* typical levels, and the typical cortical distinction between audition and vision is altered. So, even with this seemingly simple example of a classic double dissociation, things become less clearcut as we move from the sensory surface up into the neocortex.

The double dissociation method can also be applied to neuroimaging results from typical participants. If a given task activates one brain area but not another, and a second task produces the opposite pattern, again a similar inference is made, namely that each of the contrasting brain areas serves an independent localized function or module.

Let us review previous discussions of double dissociation, beginning with Teuber (1955), who introduced the term "double dissociation," and relate the issues that arise to criticisms of this method. It is instructive to see how Teuber talks about double dissociation in the 1955 chapter on physiological psychology in the *Annual Review of Psychology*. He does not

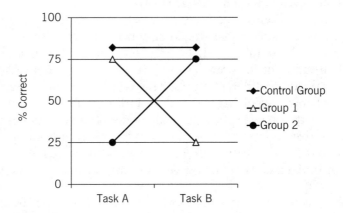

FIGURE 3.1. A double dissociation.

present a "logic of double dissociation" that specifies what inferences it permits or does not permit, nor does he advocate its use as a method to discover independent functions. Instead, he uses the term to refer to an experimental control procedure that is missing in some studies and present in others.

Even when a double dissociation is noted, Teuber is circumspect about the implications that can be drawn. In discussing a particular double dissociation, and the correlated lesions' locations, he allows that it indicates "some specificity of function," but he goes on to mention other complex tasks that are equally impaired by lesions in either of the same locations. His overall conclusion is as follows: "Such nondifferential failure speaks for generality in the effects of lesions in so-called associative cortex. Whether to stress the specific or non-specific changes is, at this stage, largely a matter of personal preference" (p. 281). In short, Teuber was *not* advocating the use of double dissociations to find independent components or modules in the cognitive architecture. Additionally, an overall concern in his review is the danger of inferring missing functions from symptoms, which is one key to the critique provided here and to a similar point made in 1864 by Hughlings Jackson: "To locate the damage which destroys speech and to localize speech are two different things" (cited in Head, 1926, p. 50).

Detailed discussions of double dissociation logic have also been provided by Shallice (1979, 1988) and Weiskrantz (1968). I will review Weiskrantz's discussion first. Like Teuber, Weiskrantz emphasizes that the "double dissociation paradigm is simply a way of combining two control procedures into a single pattern" (p. 419). He goes beyond Teuber's discussion, however, and carefully clarifies the logical limits on what can be inferred from a double dissociation (nonetheless accepting the a priori assumption that explanations should be couched in terms of independent components). Most important, he argues that a double dissociation is logically insufficient for drawing the inference that different lesions are having qualitatively different effects. This possibility is illustrated in Figure 3.2, where Group 1 has a Task A > Task B performance profile and Group 2 has the opposite, but the apparent double dissociation is not due to a qualitative difference in the effects of lesions in each group. Instead it is due to the lesions in each group affecting a cognitive resource that is shared by both tasks. We will now consider this possible scenario in more detail.

Let us assume each task in this example actually depends in part on a common cognitive resource, like attention or working memory, and that optimal performance on each task depends on a different optimal level of that resource. Let us also assume that the performance/resource functions for each task have an inverted-U shape (like the Yerkes–Dodson law), such that optimal performance is found at the top of the inverted U. If the performance/resource functions for each task overlap but are nonidentical, then a given lesion could fix resources at a point that is optimal for one task and not the other, and a different lesion could do the opposite. Then a double dissociation would be found because of a quantitative rather than qualitative difference between the effects of two lesions, as long as the two lesions differ in their effects on resources (cf. Dunn & Kirsner, 1988). One might object that Figure 3.2 depicts a very unusual scenario because the typical relation between two cognitive tasks is linear and positively correlated, such that their bivariate distribution is normal. But the situation depicted in Figure 3.1 is also unusual, because it assumes a zero correlation between the two tasks involved in the double dissociation, at least for a subset of the population. So, the fact that virtually all cognitive tasks are positively correlated means that the finding of a pure double dissociation is a statistical anomaly. Finally, Weiskrantz also mentions the problem of "reifying a dissociation between tests into a dissociation between functions" (1968, p. 419).

In sum, these early discussions of double dissociation by Teuber (1955) and Weiskrantz (1968) are circumspect and skeptical. The double dissociation method was thought to provide better experimental control than the single dissociation method, but it was not viewed as guaranteeing inferences of independent functions.

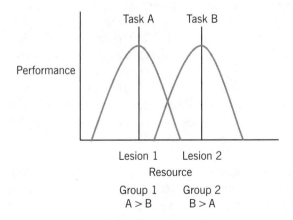

FIGURE 3.2. A double dissociation with a single underlying resource.

In the 1970s, with the beginnings of contemporary cognitive neuro-psychology, a much more optimistic view of double dissociation emerged. Dissociations, and especially double dissociations, were viewed as a powerful method for discovering functionally separate components in the cognitive architecture: "The crucial theoretical point is that the double dissociation does demonstrate that the two tasks make different processing demands on two or more functionally dissociable subsystems" (Shallice, 1979, p. 191). Given Morton and Patterson's (1980) model of single-word reading, Shallice predicted roughly 30 pure syndromes could arise! Of course, critics (Ellis, 1987; Lashley, 1929; Van Orden, Pennington, & Stone, 1990) have viewed such tendencies as inherently degenerative because they lead to the multiplication of syndromes and functions, and the multiplication of representations and rules (see the passage by Lashley quoted at the beginning of this chapter). At some point, even the most devoted modularity theorist will have to question the number of independent cognitive components implied.

Shallice (1979) also discusses how a double dissociation avoids the possible confound of a resource artifact and presents performance/resource functions to make this case. However, unlike Weiskrantz (1968), he assumes (perhaps unwarily) that these functions are nondecreasing (i.e., not inverted-U-shaped), and argues that the inference of two distinct functions from a double dissociation is sound. Consequently, the logical sufficiency of his argument depends critically on the shape of the performance/resource functions, a point that he later acknowledged in a footnote (p. 233) in his 1988 book.

In this later book, Shallice (1988) provided a much more detailed and reflective analysis of what can be inferred from double dissociations. He carefully considered threats to the validity of double dissociation logic, including the complications posed by individual differences, lesion-induced reorganization of functions, and resource artifacts. He also wrestled with tautologies that threaten to undermine this logic. One is the tautology involved in the notion of a pure case. The other is the implicit assumption that double dissociations can arise only within modular architectures. Because both of these issues have been central to the arguments presented here, it is useful to consider closely how Shallice (1988) dealt with them.

Shallice (1988) traced the notion of a pure case to Lichtheim's (1885) classic paper on subtypes of aphasia, and acknowledged what Lichtheim's critics, such as Head (1926), had implied: There is no theory-independent way of determining whether a given case is pure or mixed. Therefore the notion of what constitutes a single component (or function) depends entirely on the cognitive theory in question. Shallice argued, however, that this is not a problem for testing neuropsychological theories using single cases, because two competing theories can each produce their own set of pure cases. It can then be determined which theory best accounts for all the cases. Of course, this possibility assumes that theories will all agree on which cases are pure. But the evidential criteria that define a pure case are derived from the theory in question. Theories with different axiomatic assumptions yield different evidential criteria and different pure cases.

Moreover, there are really two tautologies embedded in the concept of pure cases. The first is the one just discussed: Different theories will pick different pure cases. The second tautology acknowledged by Shallice (1988) is more subtle. The notion of a pure case itself, regardless of which particular components are counted as independent, derives from the assumption that there *are* truly independent components to be found in behavior. In other words, the notion of a pure case must assume, a priori, that the modularity hypothesis is true. Because of this second tautology, pure cases cannot establish the validity of the modularity hypotheses.

After revealing this fallacy, Shallice went on to consider possible non-modular architectures that might produce double dissociations, including a multilevel neural network (see Chapter 4). A multilevel neural network was first explored by Wood (1978, 1982) to question the inferences from dissociations. Shallice (1988) criticized this work and then made the strong claim that it was most unlikely "that a classical or strong double dissociation can be demonstrated in a properly distributed memory system" (p. 256). He went on to replace the concept of functionally isolable systems with that of functional specialization of a *part* of a system (essentially, an unspecified component of a component). He argued that the inference of functional specializations from a double dissociation still holds, given (1) such components exist (a tautology) and (2) their absence is directly (transparently) reflected in behavior after a lesion (which does not hold for an interdependent system). So for Shallice (1988) the debate over the validity of the double dissociation method came down to whether a multilevel neural network could exhibit a double dissociation.

Subsequently, there have been numerous demonstrations that such networks can demonstrate double dissociations, and some of these demonstrations were by Shallice himself and his collaborators (Hinton & Shallice, 1991, discussed in more detail in Chapter 5; Plaut & Shallice, 1993). These demonstrations have mainly been in models of single-word reading, in which double dissociations between different groups of people with acquired dyslexia had been used by reading researchers (e.g.,

Coltheart, 1989; Morton & Patterson, 1980) to argue for a dual-route model of pronouncing single printed words. In such models, each route is considered to be an independent cognitive component or module, such that each route or component can be selectively damaged. So, for instance, one might observe contrasting dissociations across patients for reading concrete versus abstract words or for reading pseudowords versus irregular words, and infer separate cognitive components for each kind of word reading. Four studies that used connectionist models (Hinton & Shallice, 1991; Plaut, 1995, 2002; Plaut & Shallice, 1993) demonstrated how the first double dissociation (between concrete versus abstract word reading) could arise from different types of damage to the same neural network. Other studies with connectionist networks demonstrated how the second double dissociation (between pseudoword versus irregular word reading) could also arise in such a network (Harm & Seidenberg, 1999, 2004). So, different parts of the same interactive network become somewhat specialized for different aspects of the task at hand (e.g., pronouncing different kinds of single words or pseudowords), such that damage to different parts of the same network can produce an apparent double dissociation. But the mapping between behavior and aspects of the network's structure is not transparent as modular theories assert, and the dissociations are usually partial rather than completely selective. For instance, a perturbation of the network that differentially impairs pseudoword reading over irregular word reading nonetheless impairs irregular word reading to some extent (and vice versa). In sum, in this latest round of the localization debate, the connectionist critique of the method of double dissociation makes clear why this method does not work as intended.

STRUCTURAL AND FUNCTIONAL NETWORKS

The connectionist neural network models discussed here and in more detail in Chapter 4 are mathematical models of brain function, so it is important to test whether such networks actually exist in the brain. Empirical support for such networks has come later, with the advent of more sophisticated neuroimaging methods for measuring structural and functional connectivity in the brain. Structural connectivity refers to white-matter connections in the brain, which are measured by diffusion tensor imaging (DTI) using a structural MRI scan. Functional connectivity refers to patterns of correlated activity between voxels in the brain as measured by fMRI. In both cases, sophisticated mathematical methods have emerged that allow the structural or functional connectivity of the entire brain to be determined. One such very useful mathematical method is called "graph analysis" (Sporns & Zwi, 2004). In this method, each voxel is a point on a two-dimensional graph and each significant structural or functional connection between a pair of voxels is a path, leading to an overall diagram or graph of the connectivity of the brain. Using this method, it has been discovered that the adult human brain exhibits a "small world" pattern of connectivity, that is, a number of small local networks, each with dense interconnections, and a sparser pattern of connections among local networks. Graph analysis has also been applied to typical human brain development, individual differences in intelligence, and to psychopathologies like autism and schizophrenia (Menon, 2011). Some of this work will be discussed later. What is important to note here is that such connectivity analyses represent an important conceptual alternative to a traditional localizationist approach for understanding brain–behavior relations.

CHAPTER SUMMARY

We have reviewed the problems in both classical and contemporary arguments for localization of function. Round 5 helps clarify why, until recently, this issue has been so difficult to settle. As noted, theoretically plausible, formal alternatives to localizationist accounts have only recently become available. More subtly, "localization of function" embeds several assumptions espoused by different localizationists to different degrees. Indeed, successive recurrences of the localization debate tended to focus on different embedded assumptions, although a core axis of the debate is always holism versus reductionism.

These assumptions include the a priori assumption of independent functions and the two tautologies embedded in the concept of pure cases (the definition of a pure case is theory dependent and the notion of a pure case presupposes that independent functions exist). We have seen that the main contemporary method for localizing functions, double dissociation, using either lesion or neuroimaging data, is flawed.

Since any explanation of abnormal function depends on a theory of normal function, early neurologists were hampered by the lack of theories of normal function and behavioral tests of those functions. They knew about the macroanatomy of the brain, which the pioneering dissections of Vesalius and Willis had provided some centuries earlier. But they knew nothing of the microstructure of the brain. In other words, they accepted the brain hypothesis but had no knowledge of the neuron hypothesis (the idea, first advocated by Ramón y Cajal, that the brain is composed of individual cells, i.e., neurons). The ideal progression of science would be to have a theory of normal brain–behavior relations and then predict what would happen when a certain part of the brain was lesioned. Instead, the field advanced in the *opposite* direction, by going from the effects of lesions to models of normal function. It was also sometimes focused more on confirmation than disconfirmation. A lesion that disrupted a function showed that a certain part of the brain was necessary for the function but did not prove that it was sufficient. The behavioral changes after an acquired lesion thus had the ability to reject some hypotheses about brain—behavior relations, but these were fairly broad: dualism (i.e., mind and brain are distinct; see Chapter 2) was rejected and complete equipotentiality was rejected.

As we will see when we turn to disorders, arguments about localization of function are central to modern cognitive neuroscience, but now we can place many more constraints on those arguments. Most importantly, holist objections finally have (1) their own theoretical framework in connectionist network models and the powerful simulations they provide, and (2) an empirical method for identifying structural and functional networks in the brain. Connectionist models and studies of brain connectivity have begun to demonstrate how the brain can accomplish functions in a distributed and interactive way, and how abnormal behavior can arise from alterations in brain connectivity.

So, the foundational concept of neuropsychology, localization of function, is both beguilingly simple and probably an oxymoron. If we think about both terms in this phrase, one ("localization") seems fairly simple to define, and the other, "function," is much more elusive. In the realm of behavior, a function is something an organism does that is adaptive *in the context in which it evolved*. So, functions are always embedded in contexts and are difficult to isolate, as we explained earlier in the example of the light switch. As discussed earlier, like foundational concepts in other scientific disciplines—like the concept of a gene in biology or energy in physics—the concept of localization of function has generated many valuable findings, and in the process, the concept itself has evolved. We have learned that both genes and brain locations are part of complex networks, whose interactions we are still seeking to unravel.

We have also considered how the issue of localization relates to the issues of innateness and plasticity. While no function is strictly localized, functions do vary in their innateness and plasticity. As we consider different domains of function in Part II, we will review evidence bearing on their degree of localization, innateness, and plasticity. We will see that different brain structure–function relations vary along these three dimensions.

EXERCISE

Define "tautology." Are there modern neuropsychological practices that are tautological in nature? Hint: Consider the means of diagnosis for intellectual impairment.

CHAPTER 4

■■■■■■■■

How Does the Brain Compute?

W e now return to the fifth round of the localization debate (see Table 3.1), which finally provided both mathematical models (i.e., connectionist neural network models) and neuroanatomical findings (structural and functional connectivity) to support holistic notions of brain organization. These developments are pertinent for understanding abnormal behavior because they supported a much wider range of models for explaining abnormal behavior than the simple subtraction model discussed in the last chapter. This wider range of conceptual models is reviewed in Chapter 5 and then applied to specific examples of abnormal behavior in the remainder of the book.

As stated before, the early neurologists did not know about the microstructure of the brain. They also lacked a theory of information and computation, which was only developed in the 20th century. In this chapter, we will trace how advances in the understanding of neurons and their connections eventually joined with advances in theory of computation to provide the basis for neural network or connectionist models of brain functions. The main breakthroughs on the neural side of this eventual "marriage" between neurology and computation were (1) the establishment of the neuron doctrine by Ramón y Cajal; (2) extensive research on how neuronal physiology produces the action potential, culminating in a mathematical model of neuronal function (the McCulloch–Pitts neuron); (3) extensive research on the function of synapses; and (4) important discoveries in the last few decades about brain development and plasticity. In what follows, I will describe in more detail the development of a theory of computation and the development of neural network models.

Now let us consider in more detail what it means to compute. In the most general sense, a computation maps one domain onto another domain in a systematic way. Mathematically, we represent this mapping as a function, such as $y = f(x)$, where x and y are the two domains and f is the function that maps the x domain onto the y domain. The mapping function could be linear (i.e., y increases as x increases, so that the plot of their relation on a graph with an x and y axis will be a straight line) or nonlinear (e.g., as in Figure 3.2). As long as x and y are single-valued variables or scalars, the math we all learned in high school algebra allows us to perform these kinds of computations. Now, let us take a step up in complexity and imagine that x and y are now multivalued variables or vectors. Each particular x or y is now a point in a multidimensional space, and its value is a set of numbers specifying its location on each dimension in that space, for instance $x = <a, b, c>$ for a point in three-dimensional space with axes a, b, and c. The weighted input to the model neuron in Figure 4.1 (see page 44) is a three-valued vector. To map the domain of x onto y in this case, we need the tools of linear algebra, specifically matrix multiplication, which is discussed later.

As we will see, nervous systems are performing this kind of computation whenever they convert a sensory input into a motor output. Say we use our eyes to localize a desirable piece of food (such as an M&M) and want to pick it up. To do this, we must map the three-dimensional location of the M&M (a three-valued vector at least) onto a command for our motor system (another three-valued vector at least). Because each three-dimensional space has a different scale and shape, a fairly complex mathematical function is needed to map between the two (Churchland, 1995). But by using matrix multiplication embodied in weighted connections between neurons, the brain can accomplish this computation without explicitly representing the complex mathematical function. Obviously, virtually any animal's nervous system has to compute these kinds of sensory–motor mappings. The layers of **interneurons** between the sensory input and the motor output, which exist in mammalian and avian nervous systems, allow for computation of these highly complex mappings.

Notice, too, that saying that brains compute such mappings is not equivalent to stimulus–response (S-R) behaviorism, which would imply that the external sensory stimulus and its singular response in the motor cortex are the only two components of this process. The key insight of the cognitive revolution was that there are important intermediate representations (coded by hidden units in a neural network model and neurons in secondary and tertiary areas of the neocortex) between the stimulus and the response, ones that provided a degree of abstraction to learned behavior not readily accounted for by a string of S-R associations. In the simple example above, the mapping function between visual and motor space is such a representation, one that would allow the animal to make predictions about novel food locations it had never encountered before. Although Tolman (1948) found early evidence that rodents formed such abstract cognitive maps (internal representations), it took several decades before the behavioristic paradigm was overturned in psychology. Abstract mental representations (like concepts, rules, theories, etc.) are key to explaining many aspects of human and animal behavior. Neural network models are capable of learning such abstract representations, and thus can provide a way of implementing cognitive theories that models using simple S-R associations cannot.

Describing the kinds of computations that brains must perform in formal mathematical terms, like matrix multiplication, does not commit us to an explanation of *how* brains perform these calculations. The brain could be an analog computer like a slide rule or abacus or it could be a symbolic computer like your laptop, or it could be something else. Tracing the history of theories of computation in the 20th century (see Table 4.1) shows us what that something else could be.

The story of theories of computation begins with developments in the foundations of mathematics that began in the late 19th century. Mathematicians wished to place all of mathematics in a formal system, similar to Euclid's axioms for geometry. In such a system, the axioms are the "primitives" or accepted propositions, and from them various theorems can be derived by applying permissible logical operations. Hilbert and others pursued this project, and in 1900 Bertrand Russell and Albert North Whitehead published *Principia Mathematica*, which provided an axiomatic treatment of mathematics (Whitehead & Russell, 1912). Russell and Whitehead discovered an important problem that threatened the viability of this project, which was that certain possible propositions were indeterminable in their truth value. For instance, if there is a set of all sets, does it include itself as a member? They were unable to solve this problem, raising the possibility that a complete formal treatment of mathematics might be impossible. Kurt Gödel (1931) confirmed this possibility for an axiomatic system rich enough to support arithmetic, by demonstrating that such a system could generate self-referential theorems that were either undecidable or inconsistent. Some later writers (e.g., Hofstader, 1980) have taken Gödel's theorem to set an absolute limit on a scientific psychology, since an axiomatic system rich enough to generate human behavior would have to be more complicated than one for arithmetic.

Nonetheless, this work on the foundations of mathematics provided insights about mechanical computation that informed development of

TABLE 4.1. Important Dates in the Development of Neural Networks

Around 1900	*Principia Mathematica*, by B. Russell and A. N. Whitehead (Whitehead & Russell, 1912), is published.
1931	*Incompleteness Theorem*, by K. Gödel (Gödel, 1931), is published.
1936	A. Turing describes his "Turing machine," which helped define limits of what is computable in principle by a human or a machine.
1943	McCulloch and Pitts propose a model neuron in "A Logical Calculus of the Ideas Immanent in Nervous Activity" (McCulloch & Pitts, 1943).
Late 1940s	J. von Neumann and colleagues develop the first electronic computer.
1949	D. O. Hebb proposes neuronal cell assemblies and a learning rule (Hebb, 1949).
1960	F. Rosenblatt studies perceptrons and Widrow and Hoff study adalines; both perceptrons and adalines are two-layer neural networks (Rosenblatt, 1960; Widrow & Hoff, 1960).
1962	Rosenblatt proves that his learning algorithm for two-layer nets will converge on an optimal solution.
1969	*Perceptrons* by Minsky and Papert proves that a two-layer net cannot solve the XOR problem; they admit a three-layer net could solve XOR, but no learning algorithm is known for a three-layer net and they argue one will never be found. Therefore, neural network simulations of human cognition are necessarily quite limited (Minsky & Papert, 1969).
1970s	Associative, content-addressable memories developed by Anderson, Willshaw, Marr, and Kohonen.
1974	P. Werbos develops the back-propagation algorithm in his doctoral dissertation, which provides a learning algorithm for three-layer nets.
Early 1980s	D. E. Rumelhart and D. B. Parker independently rediscover the back-propagation algorithm. G. Hinton and T. Sejnowski (1986) develop the Boltzmann machine learning procedure, a form of unsupervised learning similar to Hebbian learning.
1986	*Parellel Distributed Processing* volumes are published by Rumelhart, McClelland, and the PDP Group (Rumelhart & McClelland, 1986).
1989	Hornik, Stinchcombe, and White (1989) prove that the class of three-layer networks constitutes a universal function approximator. Siegelmann (1999) proves that the networks in this class are equivalent to a Turing machine; therefore, they have the same computational power as a symbolic computer.

the first electronic computer by Allen Turing and John von Neumann. In the idealized Turing machine and in actual electronic computers used today, the form of computation is essentially that used in symbolic logic: symbolic propositions are inputs and are transformed through a series of rule-governed steps into output propositions. Hence, carrying out a given computation involves many iterative steps until the program reaches its specified end state. But since information flows at essentially the speed of light in an electronic computer, these many steps could still be accomplished very quickly. As everyone knows, this form of mechanical computation has been enormously successful but, for reasons discussed below, is unlikely to be the correct model for neural computations. Even so, the formal systems developed by mathematicians and instantiated in symbolic computers became the root metaphor for early cognitive scientists, among them Noam Chomsky and Jean Piaget. For Chomsky, the "deep structure" of language was an innate formal system capable of generating the infinite number of syntactically legal sentences (propositions) a human can produce. For Piaget, these formal structures of cognition developed through interaction with experience, with simpler logical operations being replaced by more powerful ones, eventuating in a mature logical system that Piaget called "formal operations." Both of these pioneers in the cognitive revolution understood that human brains must perform computations, and they took as their model for how that was done the theory of computation that was available at that time. The same computer metaphor of human cognition was at the heart of later developments in cognitive psychology, such as the simulations of problem solving by Newell and Simon (1972), production systems developed by Anderson (1983) and in work on artificial intelligence (AI).

But a different line of thinking about the human brain's computation was being pursued at the same time. As we saw earlier, this line of thinking began with an idealized neuron proposed by McCulloch and Pitts (1943). Figure 4.1 displays this model neuron. The key features of this neuron are (1) weighted inputs from other neurons onto the dendrites on the left of the figure; (2) a method for integrating these weighted inputs

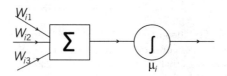

FIGURE 4.1. McCulloch and Pitts's ideal neuron.

in the neuronal cell body (the summation sign in the square); and (3) a threshold function for determining whether the neuron fires or not (the step function in the circle on the right). Neuronal firing is generally all or none, and whether a neuron fires or not is a function of all the inputs it is receiving at that time. The threshold function is a mathematical function that describes the relation between the continuous summed input to a neuron and its dichotomous output (i.e., firing or not firing). Because each neuron is essentially acting as a signal detector, its accuracy will be improved if the threshold function is nonlinear (e.g., a step function or a sigmoid function as shown in Figure 4.1). Hence, one can think of a single neuron as implementing a low-level form of categorical perception, which is discussed in Chapters 6 and 8.

If the neuron fires, an action potential is propagated down the axon on the right, and this axon and its collaterals have multiple connections (synapses) on the dendrites of other neurons (not shown). In this model, the three weighted lines feeding into the square are dendrites that provide inputs from other neurons to these neurons. When one of those input neurons "fires," its input signal is weighted by the connection strength (W_i) of its synapse on the dendrite. Although the neuron in the model has only three input connections, a typical real neuron in the human brain has 10^5 input connections. In the model, the three weighted inputs are added up (summation sign, Σ) in the neuronal cell body, and that net input is passed to a threshold function in the circle. If the net input crosses the threshold, then the neuron fires an action potential down its axon, which reaches the dendrites of many other downstream neurons (because the axon branches into many collaterals). So the individual neuron is a "detector" that fires when it receives a certain amount of input. It is important to notice that the decision to fire is nonlinear, because the threshold function is not linear (in Figure 4.1 it is a step function). The individual model neuron is performing a simple computation: it is mapping an input pattern onto an output pattern. So, the science of neuronal functioning captured in this model neuron revealed that neurons were nonlinear signal integrators or detectors. Could a network composed of such model neurons perform useful computations? As we will see, the answer turned out to be "yes," but several intermediate questions had to be answered before this outcome was reached.

A key intermediate question was how such neural circuits could learn. Hebb (1949) proposed a very simple learning rule, namely that "neurons that fire together, wire together." In other words, if both the pre- and postsynaptic neurons were firing at the same time, the synaptic connection between them would be strengthened. Although Hebb did not know what the mechanism of this synaptic modification was, and he did not quantify his learning rule, his insight was profound, and the molecular details of Hebbian learning have since been worked out.

In the 1960s, Rosenblatt (1960) and others tested the computational limits of a McCulloch–Pitts neuron with a two-layer neural network called a *perceptron*. The first layer was simply an input layer (on which the vector for a particular input pattern could be represented), and the second layer was the model neuron itself. There were connections from each input unit to each weighted dendrite in the model neuron (imagine multiple connections to each line on the left of Figure 4.1). Rosenblatt developed a learning rule for the perceptron and proved mathematically that it would converge on an optimal solution for learning an input–output mapping.

There was considerable resistance to Rosenblatt's approach by proponents of symbolic AI and the dominant computer metaphor of the human mind. Minsky and Papert (1969) published a very influential critique of the computational properties of perceptrons. They proved that perceptrons could not solve the exclusive OR (XOR) problem, which humans obviously can. XOR is a logical function that says the system should respond when either input A or B is present, but *not both* A and B. Going back to the light switch analogy in Chapter 1, we can provide an everyday example of the XOR function. It can be found in many houses when there are two light switches in different parts of a room controlling a single light. The light will come on if only *one* switch is turned on, but not both. So, this logical function combines the simpler inclusive OR function (either A or B; or both A and B) with a negation of the latter AND function (both A and B). One can see that the XOR function is not additive and thus more complex than the inclusive OR or AND. Minksy and Papert (1969) acknowledged that XOR could be solved by a three-layer perceptron, with one layer performing the inclusive OR function and the second layer performing the negation of the AND function, but they argued that a learning algorithm for a three layer neural network would never be found (a weak argument because it hinges on predicting the future). Hence, they maintained that this approach to modeling human cognition was limited to very simple pattern recognition problems.

In the 1970s, other cognitive psychologists (Anderson, 1983; Kohonen, 1984; Marr, 1970; Willshaw, 1972) used perceptron-based architectures to develop associative, content-addressable memory simulations. This was important because human memory is content-addressable, not location-addressable like the memory of a symbolic computer. If I am trying to remember a conversation or someone's name, I use the context of the conversation or other things I know about the person to guide my memory search. In other words, because related contents are connected in my memory, I can use contents I remember to help me search for other contents I cannot spontaneously recall. I definitely do not command the internal librarian to go to row X and shelf Y. Thus, perceptron-based architectures were relevant and plentiful in cognitive psychology.

Just 5 years after Minsky and Papert (1969) proclaimed that a learning algorithm for a three-layer network was impossible, Paul Werbos (1974) developed one in his unpublished doctoral dissertation at Harvard. In the early 1980s, two mathematical psychologists, David Rumelhart and D. B. Parker, independently developed the same back-propagation algorithm for supervised learning in a three-layer network. Using this learning algorithm, a three-layer network *could* solve the XOR problem that Minsky and Papert (1969) had proclaimed would never be solved by a neural network model. Around the same time, Hinton and Sejnowksi (1986) developed the Boltzmann machine learning procedure, a form of unsupervised learning similar to Hebbian learning. These two learning algorithms, one requiring an external "teacher" and the other not, permitted wide application of connectionist networks to the simulation of human cognition and began a scientific revolution that is still unfolding today. In 1986, Rumelhart, McClelland, and colleagues published the classic two-volume book *Parallel Distributed Processing*, which explained this new approach to simulating human cognition (Rumelhart & McClelland, 1986). In 1989, Hornik, Stinchcombe, and White (1989) proved mathematically that the class of three-layer neural networks constitutes a universal function approximator. Ten years later, Siegelmann (1999) proved that this class of networks is computationally equivalent to a Turing machine, meaning they have the same computational power as a symbolic computer (Hornik et al., 1989).

So, what are some reasons for preferring connectionist over symbolic computation for what human brains actually do? Table 4.2 lists some of the reasons. A very important reason is the consilience principle discussed earlier, in two ways. First, in the time a human brain performs a complex computation, it could not have transmitted neural impulses fast enough to execute the multiple serial processing steps needed by a symbolic computer to perform the same computation. Second, connectionist computation is consistent with the function of individual neurons and groups of neurons. As explained at the beginning of this chapter, the kind of computation that brains perform involves matrix multiplication; neurons and groups of neurons are perfect for performing this kind of computation (Figure 4.2).

In Figure 4.2, we now have three idealized neurons (p, q, and r), each receiving the same four-valued vector ($<a, b, c, d>$) on its dendrites. Each

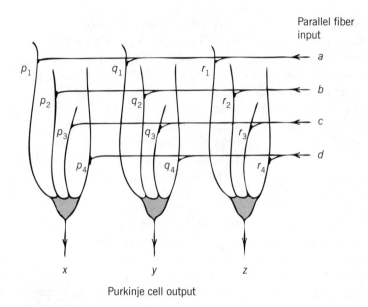

FIGURE 4.2. A simple neural network. From Churchland (1986, p. 429). Copyright 1986 by The Massachusetts Institute of Technology. Reprinted by permission.

neuron weights these inputs differently (each has four weights, denoted by p_1–p_4, q_1–q_4, and r_1–r_4 in the figure). The weighted inputs are summed in each neuronal cell body and passed through a threshold function, which determines whether the individual neuron fires or not. The firing pattern of the three neurons produces an output vector, $<x, y, z>$. So the three neurons compute a mapping between the input vector and the output vector through matrix multiplication. The weight matrix that accomplishes this is a 4-by-3 matrix (four weights on each of three neurons). So this simple neural network converts a four-valued input vector into a three-valued output vector. As we increase the number of neurons and connections, the dimensionality (complexity) of the information represented increases. With 10^5 inputs to each of the 10^{10} neurons in a human brain, the number of possible informational states our brain can take on is vast.

Table 4.2 lists other advantages to a connectionist approach to brain computation discussed by Smolensky (Smolensky & D'Alonzo, 1988). One is that such networks learn and develop based on input from the environment, as we know human children and other developing animals do. So neural network models are consistent with what we know about

TABLE 4.2. Implications of Connectionism

1. Consistent with brain structure and brain development.
2. Simulates learning and development—provides an explanation of sensitive periods and stages.
3. Deals nicely with problem of partial knowledge.
4. Deals nicely with problem of learning quasi-regular domains of knowledge, such as past-tense or printed word recognition in languages like English. Shows how we can capture both rule-like regularities and context-sensitive irregularities with the same computational mechanism.
5. Models top-down effects, such as the word superiority effect.
6. Can simulate normal development, atypical development, and loss of function due to brain damage in one network.

brain plasticity and its role in development. It is hard to imagine how a symbolic computer program could be incrementally modified by such environmental input and keep functioning. Also, like human children, such networks exhibit partial knowledge. They can learn part of a rule or regularity and still function, whereas it is hard to imagine how a symbolic computer could learn part of a rule. Another advantage is that much of what humans learn is quasi-regular, and context sensitive, whether it be the past-tense forms of English words or category membership (e.g., is something a game or not?). A symbolic computer approaches such a learning problem by having a few invariant rules and then a case-by-case memory for the many exceptions. Such networks, if they have bidirectional connections between layers, as the human brain has, can easily simulate top-down effects on processing, which is another important example of context sensitivity. The sixth reason on the list in Table 4.2 is the thesis of this book, which is that connectionist networks provide a common framework for simulating normal development, developmental disorders, and acquired disorders.

Next we will consider an early, simple neural network model and discuss how it bears on the issue of localization of function. This example is the interactive-activation model of the **word superiority effect** developed by McClelland and Rumelhart (1981). Their model illustrates how top-down influences affect language processing. The word superiority effect arises in an experimental paradigm in which the participant sees briefly presented letter strings, either real words (e.g., "trip") or nonwords (e.g., "pirt"), or a single letter ("t"), and then makes a forced-choice decision about which letter he or she saw (e.g., a "t" or a "k"). There is a robust accuracy advantage for real words versus nonwords and, surprisingly, for both real words and nonwords versus single letters. Such an effect was puzzling given the widely assumed unidirectional information processing model prevalent at the time, since letter identification was thought to be complete before the stage of word identification began. So participants were expected to perform equally on probe letters following real words and nonwords, and *better* on individual letters.

In their influential early connectionist style model (the **interactive activation model**), McClelland and Rumelhart (1981; Rumelhart & McClelland, 1982) demonstrated how top-down feedback connections from the lexical level could activate or inhibit individual letter representations and thus account for the word superiority effect. In other words, letter identification was *not* complete before lexical processing began, as a strict unidirectional processing model requires. If processing were unidirectional, single letters would be easiest to identify and real words and nonwords would be less so (because there are more individual letters to consider). Since top-down effects are pervasive in language processing, as many studies have documented, then localizing discrete stages of language processing in the brain is much more difficult, if not impossible. That is because the activity observed at a layer or hub in the brain's neural network will be due to several things: (1) bottom-up input; (2) the particular computation that layer performs; and (3) top-down input, which biases that layer's computation. This recurrent interaction between different layers in the network blurs the distinct contributions of any one of them, such that the resulting brain activity we observe with neuroimaging methods is hard to parse apart. Many imaging studies have attempted to localize components of language processing, and the results sometimes conform to classical language models (e.g., syntax is more anterior than posterior), but there have been many conflicting results.

Finally, because of brain plasticity, it is important to realize that localization of functions, especially in the neocortex, can change with development, and the connectionist networks can easily accommodate this fact of development. Mark Johnson and Michelle de Haan (2006) call this process of changing localization "**interactive specialization.**" This term means that the functional specializations of the human neocortex emerge as a result of a developmental process in which *interactions* among components of a functional brain network determine the changing role of each participating brain area. They contrast their interactive specialization theory with a maturational model of brain development, such as Fodor's (1983) modularity theory, in which the functional specialization of a given neocortical region is innately determined. As we will see, for many (but not all) neocortical functions, the evidence favors the interactive specialization model over the maturational one.

CHAPTER SUMMARY

Neural network models have helped resolve the most recent round in the localization of function debate by providing a detailed, more realistic account of how the brain computes than was provided by earlier box-and-arrow models. These neural network models have been applied extensively to most of the domains of function considered in Part II—perception, attention, memory, language, and executive functions (EFs)—and to disorders in those domains. So, neural network models provide an important alternative model for explaining abnormal behavior. In the next section, we consider various alternative models for explaining abnormal behavior at a *conceptual* level. Then in subsequent chapters we review how these models can be applied to actual examples of abnormal behavior.

CHAPTER 5

■■■■■■■

Classical and Contemporary Models of Abnormal Behavior

As we saw in Chapter 3, the field of neuropsychology began in the early 19th century with the phrenological studies of Gall and Spurzheim, followed by discoveries by Broca, Wernicke, and others that demonstrated that localized damage in the adult human left hemisphere could disrupt language functions. These discoveries led to *four* classical models of how acquired brain damage disrupts function and spurred debates that continue today regarding the seemingly innocuous concept of "localization of function." In what follows, I first describe and critique these four classical models, and then describe contemporary models. The overall goal of this chapter is to examine which models are most useful for a unified theory of abnormal behavior across the fields of neurology, psychiatry, and developmental disorders.

SUBTRACTION

In Chapter 3, we have already provided an extensive critique of the subtraction model, which conceptually is the simplest and most straightforward model of how brain damage disrupts function. Because of its simplicity, it is not surprising that early neurologists first turned to the subtraction model to explain the behavioral effects of acquired lesions. Returning to what was said in Chapter 3, the subtraction model posits that functions such as language are localized in the adult brain, and that damage to a localized center for a function *selectively* degrades or eliminates that function, leaving other functions intact, such that mapping between brain and behavior is *transparent*. While this simple model is possible, especially for low-level sensory disorders (e.g., a visual field cut caused by severing some of the optic pathways in the brain) and may hold true for some higher-level disorders discussed later (e.g., hippocampal amnesia), there are several issues with the logic of the subtraction model that we have discussed earlier and will review here. First, as we discussed in the example of the light switch in Chapter 1, loss of function after a focal brain lesion only demonstrates that the lesioned region is *necessary* for the lost function, but not sufficient for that function. What are the other assumptions of the subtraction model and how valid are they? As discussed in the previous sections on the localization debate and double dissociation logic, the subtraction model assumes that functions are independent. This assumption means that the brain is a mosaic of different functionally separate complex functions, such that localized damage can degrade or eliminate one function while leaving the rest intact. This assumption is called the assumption of **pure insertion** (or we could say "pure subtraction") and has a long history in experimental psychology, going back to Donders. It is also a key and contentious assumption in contemporary functional neuroimaging studies. The key flaw in the independence or pure insertion assumption is that it does not address how different functions in the brain are integrated to produce coherent action.

DISCONNECTION

This model was first described by Wernicke after his discovery of a patient whose speech was fluent and language comprehension intact, but who was very impaired in the ability to repeat speech. On autopsy, Wernicke discovered that this patient had damage to the white matter tract (the arcuate fasciculus) connecting Wernicke's area to Broca's area. So, not only were there at least *two* language centers instead of one, but these centers were connected to each other, suggesting their functions were connected as well. This third kind of aphasia was termed **conduction aphasia** because it involved damage to the pathway that conducted information from Wernicke's area to Broca's area. Conduction aphasia was the first example of what has come to be known as a "disconnection syndrome." As we will see later in the book, disconnection as a theoretical model continues to be very important in contemporary accounts of neurodevelopmental disorders such as dyslexia and autism, and we will return to modern methods for analyzing brain connectivity later in this chapter.

The theoretical model that Wernicke elaborated in his dissertation to explain these three kinds of aphasia involved both centers as well as the connections between them. In his model, there were two localized main language functions, comprehension and speech production (input and output processing), and the connection between them. Disconnection left these two main language functions intact but prevented them from inter-acting. So speech input could be comprehended, but it could not reach the output center to allow repetition. The important point here is that the disconnection model is a rival hypothesis to the subtraction model. If a patient has lost a normal function, it may be due to disconnection rather than damage to the localized center for that function.

There are some further assumptions in Wernicke's use of disconnec-tion that have not proven valid. Wernicke's model of the two language centers and their connection was a "boxes-and-arrows" model of the sort that typified early information processing theories in the 20th century, and it made some of the same assumptions later identified as problems in those models. It retained the assumption of pure insertion found in the subtraction model, even though the functions that were individuated were components of the very broad functions assumed by the phrenologists. A key second assumption was that connections (arrows) were unidirec-tional: information flow went from input to output, but output centers did not project back to input centers. Only in the second half of the 20th century did anatomical and functional discoveries make it clear that infor-mation flow in the brain was *bidirectional*.

MULTIPLE DEFICITS

Later 19th-century neurologists elaborated Wernicke's model (Figure 8.3), adding other centers and connections to account for patients with acquired lesion who had different profiles of functional deficits. For instance, Lich-theim added a semantic center and Dejerine added a word-reading center. Dejerine also described a patient with a curious symptom profile, alexia without agraphia, meaning the patient could write a message but could not read his own message or those of others. Since writing and reading seem to have many components in common, how could such a symptom profile arise? On autopsy, Dejerine found this patient had *two* lesions, one to the primary visual area (V1) in the left hemisphere and a second to the posterior portion of the corpus callosum (called the splenium), which connects the posterior left and right hemispheres. Dejerine's expla-nation of the patient's symptom profile combined the first two models just discussed, subtraction and disconnection. The left-hemisphere lesion in V1 *subtracted* visual input on that side of the brain, but the patient was not blind because V1 in the right hemisphere was intact. The splenium lesion *disconnected* visual input from the right hemisphere to the language center in the posterior left-hemisphere angular gyrus, impairing reading. But because the left hemisphere language centers were all intact independently, the patient had normal spoken language and writing. The result is a multiple deficit model with a symptom profile that is produced by the combination of two lesions and two resulting deficits.

A modern application of the multiple deficit model can be found in a connectionist model of the puzzling acquired neurological syndrome of optic aphasia (Sitton, Mozer, & Farah, 2000). Patients with this syndrome are impaired at naming pictures but do not have apperceptive visual agnosia (inability to recognize pictures) or a generalized anomia (inability to retrieve names with or without pictures). (Apperceptive visual agnosia is discussed in more detail in Chapter 6.) Unlike anomic patients, these patients can name objects when given a verbal definition or can act out the meaning of a visually presented object. Unlike agnosics, they can hone in on the correct name for a picture through an effortful process of generating the names of semantically related objects, and their recognition of visual objects is not affected by the visual quality of the stimulus. So, what makes optic aphasia puzzling to explain is that all the components (i.e., visual perception, semantics, and naming, as well as the connections between them) required for picture naming appear to be intact, yet patients with optic aphasia are impaired at it. The traditional solution to this kind of puzzle is to maintain the assumption that there is a single neurological cause (damage to a single center or route), and then to add more boxes and arrows to the model, such that a single lesion will reproduce the behavior in question. However, this solution to the puzzle risks being ad hoc and is less parsimonious than a solution with fewer processing components. Instead, Sitton et al. (2000) proposed that the superadditive interaction between *two* partial disconnections (between visual perception and semantics and between semantics and naming) could produce the profile of impaired and intact behavior observed in optic aphasia. They created a connectionist model of visual object naming to test this hypothesis and found that the interactive effects of these two partial disconnections could reproduce the entire symptom profile. (But see Plaut, 2002, for a single-lesion explanation of optic apahasia.)

The move from single to multiple deficits to explain abnormal behavior acknowledges both the interactivity of the brain and the likely multifactorial basis of many disorders. As we will see in later chapters, a multiple deficit model has proved to be important in explaining some neurodevel-opmental disorders where a single localized lesion is quite unlikely.

IMBALANCE

So far, these classical models have provided different ways to explain *loss* of function, either through subtraction, disconnection, or the combination of the two. One of the greatest 19th-century behavioral neurologists, James Hughlings Jackson, was an important critic of these models, and one of his objections was that brain damage does not always simply produce *loss* of function. Instead, it sometimes produces *new* abnormal behaviors. Jackson called these new abnormal behaviors that emerge after brain damage "positive symptoms" and contrasted them to "negative symptoms," which were the loss of normal behaviors. Jackson's model for explaining positive symptoms is essentially disinhibition: brain damage can release impulses from inhibition. We call this model *imbalance* because the positive symptoms result from an imbalance between bottom-up impulses and top-down control (vertical imbalance). As we will see in subsequent chapters, the imbalance model is the main model for explaining psychiatric disorders such as mood disorders, action selection disorders like Tourette syndrome, and aspects of schizophrenia. As will be discussed in Chapter 11, a different horizontal imbalance model is also sometimes used to explain positive symptoms (such as the tics in Tourette syndrome).

The imbalance model is less static than the subtraction and disconnection models because it asserts there is a dynamic interaction between different parts of the brain and a balance between opponent processes. Examples of positive symptoms have been used by later researchers to criticize the idea of localization of function. Gregory (1961) pointed out that diagnosing the cause of dysfunction when any complex machine stops working is very difficult because we cannot always reason backwards from the dysfunction to the responsible component in the broken machine (we all face this dilemma when our car or computer malfunctions and various repair people offer competing explanations for the problem). Gregory (1968) gave the example of a radio that begins to hum after a resistor is removed. The radio now has a positive symptom in Jackson's terms. But we would go astray if we reasoned that the function of the absent resistor is a "hum suppressor." Another example of a positive symptom is provided by the syndrome of hemiballism in rodents. After a unilateral lesion to the basal ganglia (BG), the rodent begins to run in circles. Again we would not infer that the damaged side of the BG has the function of inhibiting running in circles. Instead, we should infer that horizontal imbalance between the two sides of the BG leads to the emergence of a positive symptom.

ABNORMAL PLASTICITY

Unlike the four classical models, the three contemporary models that follow incorporate development into their explanations of abnormal behavior. Plasticity is a mechanism of brain development and refers to the ability of the brain to change its connections, either in response to the environment or in response to injury to the brain itself. Plasticity after an acquired lesion is another complication for the subtraction model because patients are usually studied after the acute phase of their brain illness and thus reorganization of functions may have occurred.

Perhaps the two best-known examples of abnormal plasticity are phantom phenomena and synesthesia. Both of these count as positive symptoms in Jackson's terms, but they do not result from imbalance. In phantom phenomena, the patient experiences sensations from a lost limb or damaged or missing sense organ. On the face of it, phantom phenomena challenge our everyday understanding of how sensations work, which is that sensations such as pain, sights, or sounds are direct experiences of external reality, not constructions or simulations produced by our mind. So, how can sensations without an external source (phantoms) arise? The best-studied case is **phantom limb pain**. The basic idea is that even though the limb is missing, its somatosensory map still exists in the brain and can be stimulated in various new ways because of plasticity, thus leading to phantom limb pain. Flor et al. (1995), using magnetoencephalography (MEG), documented reorganization of primary somatosensory cortex in patients with phantom limb pain, showing that the maps of body parts (e.g., the face) adjacent to the map of the missing limb now overlapped with it. Ramachandran (2011) provided further evidence for this plasticity explanation. He hypothesized that phantom limb pain could arise in somatosensory cortex in two ways: (1) persistent firing of the somatosensory map of the missing body part, and (2) remapping of inputs to that map. The first method means that without external input, the neurons in the somatosensory map of the absent limb keep firing (perhaps because of intracortical connections) and this firing is experienced as phantom sensations. The second way means that the brain map of the absent limb now receives input from an adjacent brain map, such as that of the face.

Indeed, he and others have documented sensations in the missing hand when the cheek is stimulated and vice versa, and corresponding alterations in the somatosensory cortex representations by means of functional neuroimaging.

Phantom phenomena are found in other sensory modalities, such as hearing. Patients who have lost hearing due to inner ear hair cell damage experience distressing humming or ringing sounds without an external source, called tinnitus. Muhlnickel, Elbert, Taub, and Flor (1998) used MEG to test whether tinnitus was an auditory phantom phenomenon. They found reorganization of the tonotopic map in primary auditory cortex that correlated highly with the experience of tinnitus. Since that discovery, other studies have found evidence that tinnitus is a phantom phenomenon.

The second example of abnormal plasticity is **synesthesia** (Ramachandran, 2011), in which individuals experience multisensory perception, even though only one sensory dimension is present in the stimulus. A common form of synesthesia is perceiving certain printed numbers and letters in a different color than their actual ink color, but synesthesia can combine other sensory modalities. The experience of synesthesia has been verified by behavioral experiments and by neuroimaging. For example, a synesthete might always see the number "3" printed in black ink as being red. We can validate this experience by testing whether "3's" exhibit visual "pop-out" in a random field of digits printed in black. If they do, the time needed to identify all the "3's" in the field will be markedly faster than the time needed for other numbers. This is exactly what happens for synesthetes and only for the numbers or letters they see in color. Neuroimaging provides another test of this phenomenon because the parts of the secondary visual cortex that are important for identifying visual objects, like the number "3," are separate from the part (V4) involved in color vision. If the synesthete is actually seeing a black "3" as red, there should be additional activity in V4, and that is what occurs.

So, how does abnormal plasticity explain synesthesia? Ramachandran (2011) explains it as an example of abnormal cross-wiring, possibly genetically caused, between V4 and the nearby fusiform gyrus involved in visual object recognition. A second possibility is that this cross-wiring could arise developmentally. We know that, in infancy, various sensory areas in the brain are more interconnected than in adulthood, leading to what is called *amodal* perception by infants. With development, many of these interconnections are literally "pruned" away, leading to sensory segregation. In such pruning, synapses that are not strengthened by Hebbian learning are eventually eliminated. So, the developmental plasticity hypothesis to explain synesthesia is essentially reduced pruning of these connections among sensory areas. We do not know which of these hypotheses is correct. However, there is recent evidence that learning plays a role in some forms of synesthesia, such as seeing numbers and letters in color. Witthoft and Winawer (2013) found that the colors perceived by eleven individuals with number–color and/or letter–color synesthesia closely matched the colors found in Fisher-Price magnetic letters and numbers. All but one of their synesthetes recalled playing with these toys as children. Of course, as these authors acknowledge, many nonsynesthetes have had similar experiences with colored letter/number toys, so early learning cannot provide the complete explanation for synesthesia.

ENVIRONMENTAL DEPRIVATION

The fact that the brain is plastic means that it depends critically on environmental input to form appropriate neural circuits. We know from extensive research by Helen Neville and colleagues (Neville et al., 1997) on congenitally deaf individuals that their auditory cortex is remapped to process visual input, including visual language (such as American Sign Language). The brain's dependence on environmental input means that lack of expected inputs can lead to abnormal circuits.

One classic example of this was discovered by Hubel and Wiesel (1998) in their experiments on the effects of monocular deprivation on the development of the primary visual cortex (V1) in cats. They found that such deprivation disrupted the formation of ocular dominance columns in V1 neocortex. Each such column is responsive to input from just one eye, and left and right eye columns intermingle across V1. These columns originally receive inputs from both eyes but through a process of competition and pruning become wired up to a single eye. Segregation of input from each eye is necessary for stereoscopic vision, so monocular deprivation leads to the loss of stereopsis, even when binocular visual input is restored.

The same phenomenon is observed in human infants with a congenital cataract in one eye. Unless the cataract is removed, they too will suffer monocular deprivation and loss of stereopsis. So an important plasticity process in normal infant development is what is called **experience-expectant synaptogenesis** (Greenough, Black, & Wallace, 1987). In the months following birth, the infant's brain overproduces synapses and "expects" species-typical experiences (like binocular visual input) to prune these synapses down to a functional set. Production and tuning of synapses also occurs throughout the life span, called **experience-dependent** synaptogenesis (Greenough et al., 1987), which allows the individual to learn from experiences, some of which may be specific to him or her (e.g., a specific episodic memory).

ALTERATION OF ATTRACTOR DYNAMICS BY DIFFUSE DAMAGE

Cross-wiring and monocular deprivation are two localized examples of how altered neural connections can produce abnormal behavior, but there can be distributed examples as well. Connectionist or neural network models, like the real brain, are plastic in that their internal connections are modified by environmental input. Such networks have been used to simulate both development and loss of specific cognitive functions, like pronouncing single printed words, recognizing visual objects, and so on.

Hinton and Shallice (1991) used a neural network model of printed-word reading to model an acquired dyslexia syndrome called **deep dyslexia**. Patients with this syndrome make two characteristic reading errors. They are very poor at reading nonwords and they make semantic errors (e.g., saying "ship" for "yacht"). Traditional box-and-arrow models of this disorder postulated two deficits; damage to the component that performs letter–sound correspondences, which is necessary for pronouncing printed nonwords, and disconnection from, or damage to, a semantic store. Hinton and Shallice designed a neural network with similar components, but unlike the box and arrow schematic model, the neural network model after training could actually produce the behavior of pronouncing words and activating their meanings. The key question in their experiment was what kind of damage to the network would produce the semantic errors that are the hallmark of deep dyslexia. Contrary to the box-and-arrow formulation, they found that damage *anywhere* in the network produced semantic errors. The explanation of this surprising result was in terms of altered attractor dynamics. Attractors can be thought of as basins in the complex multidimensional space that characterizes the interactions of components of a neural network, and a given input (a printed word) can be thought of as a marble "rolling" in that space. Because the network has learned the correct mappings between inputs (printed words) and outputs (semantic features), the rolling marble starts close to the appropriate attractor basin and typically "falls" into it, producing a correct response ("ship" for *ship*). Damage anywhere in the network introduces noise into the attractor dynamics, in effect making each attractor basin more shallow, and the path of the marble more wobbly. So, now it is easier for the marble to fall into an adjacent attractor basin and thus the network produces a semantic error ("ship" for *yacht*). As we will see later, this explanation based on altered attractor dynamics has also been successfully applied to other examples of abnormal behavior, such as visual object agnosia (Farah, 1994).

Occasionally, semantic errors are also observed in developing readers, both developmental dyslexics (Johnston, 1982; Temple, 1988) and typical beginning readers (Seymour & Elder, 1986), not because they have brain damage, but because their reading network is still developing and their attractor dynamics are noisy.

ALTERATIONS IN CONNECTIVITY

As briefly mentioned in Chapter 3, in recent decades noninvasive methods have been developed to measure structural and functional connectivity in humans, and these methods have provided a new window on abnormal behavior. Structural connectivity refers to white matter tracts in the brain. These tracts can be measured and reconstructed from a structural MRI scan with diffusion tensor imaging (DTI), which was discussed in Chapter 3. The Human Connectome Project (listed in Appendix B) is a database of DTI results from many studies that allows researchers to generate connectivity maps in typical humans at different ages and in some disorders (Plate 5.1 in the color insert). Functional connectivity refers to patterns of coactivation of voxels in an fMRI scan. Graph analysis (Sporns & Zwi, 2004) is a useful method for analyzing network structure in both structural and functional connectivity data. In this method, nodes and their connections and connection strength are identified in the data, and an overall brain network is constructed. Several summary statistics can be calculated that quantify network properties, such as the degree of local and global organization. A basic finding is that human brain networks have a *small world* pattern of organization, in which small local networks are connected by longer pathways (e.g., between local networks in the posterior cortex and the prefrontal cortex). Connectivity patterns change with development, are correlated with individual differences in IQ, and differ in some disorders, such as schizophrenia (van den Heuvel, Stam, Kahn, & Hulshoff Pol, 2009).

In this model of abnormal behavior, we have come to the most global or least localized explanation. In this model, both typical and developmental and individual differences in cognition and those found in certain disorders like schizophrenia are really an emergent property of the patterns of organization across the entire cortex. Different patterns of organization will theoretically lead to different disorders.

A final notion that is used in explaining abnormal behavior is **confabulation**. Confabulation is *not* a separate model for explaining abnormal behavior, but it can be a useful adjunct to such explanations. To confabulate means to make up a story to explain some aspect of one's own behavior or experience without intending to deceive. So, confabulation is called "honest lying," and can occur in typical children and adults when they produce false memories or justify a decision. Confabulation is more often found in brain disorders, such as certain forms of amnesia, and thus confabulation *is* usually an abnormal behavior, not an explanation for abnormal behavior. But the mechanisms underlying confabulation reveal an important aspect of the normal process by which the phenomenal self is constructed. In some disorders, this normal constructive activity, acting on deficient input, sometimes produces a confabulation, which is a type of positive symptom. Confabulation alone does not provide a complete explanation for any disorder, but it can reasonably be utilized as *part* of the explanation for some disorders. So confabulation has a different status than the previous models. As in the disconnection and imbalance models, confabulation makes it clear that symptoms often arise from a dynamic interaction between damaged and normal functions.

One of the first examples of confabulation after brain damage was found in patients whose corpus callosum had been transected to relieve intractable epilepsy. When Roger Sperry and colleagues investigated individuals who had undergone this procedure, they found that the patient would deny seeing objects presented only to the left visual field, which projects to the nonverbal right hemisphere. This denial is a confabulation from the observer's point of view, but a veridical statement given the information available to the isolated left hemisphere. More dramatically, if the left hand aided the right hand in solving a puzzle, such as Block Design, the right hand would try to push the left out of the way, and the patient would make up a story for what the left hand was doing (compare this to **alien-hand syndrome**). These and other observations of split-brain patients gave rise to the view that consciousness itself could be split and that the role of the verbal left hemisphere was to rationalize our experience, that is, to produce a coherent narrative of the information available to it.

Confabulation is also found in several other neurological disorders. In anosognosia, the patient denies that a body part belongs to him or her. In Capgras syndrome, the patient claims familiar people are impostors. And in hippocampal amnesia with frontal lobe involvement, the patient produces impossible autobiographical memories ("I went with Neil Armstrong to the moon."). In anosognosia, a patient with hemispatial neglect has lost awareness of one half of the body as belonging to them. When asked about what it is, they confabulate. For example, when asked about their left leg, they may say, "someone put a log in my bed." In Capgras syndrome, one explanation is that the fusiform face area is disconnected from emotional parts of the brain that confer a feeling of familiarity. So, when the patient sees a parent, they recognize that the person looks just like their mother or father but lack the usual feeling of familiarity, so they give the confabulated explanation that the parent must be an impostor. In hippocampal amnesia with frontal lobe involvement, the patient is both unable to form and retrieve autobiographical memories and unable to critically evaluate which memories are possible ones. So, the memories that are produced are confabulations. As we will discuss later, confabulation is also relevant for understanding delusions and hallucinations that occur in schizophrenia and sometimes in other psychiatric disorders.

Confabulation is also relevant for the brain processes that continuously generate a self-representation, which is discussed in Part III. As we will see in Part II, various disorders can selectively damage inputs to this self-representation process, leading to striking alterations in the phenomenology of the self.

CHAPTER SUMMARY

A variety of neuropsychological models have been proposed to explain abnormal behavior besides the most familiar one, the subtraction mode. In Part II, we will evaluate which models best account for different abnormal behaviors. A general conclusion we will reach is that most abnormal behaviors require abnormal interactions in neural systems and not just the simple subtraction of a component part.

Of course, a complete explanation of any abnormal behavior will require multiple levels of analysis besides the neuropsychological level. These other levels include (1) etiology (genetic and environmental risk factors); (2) molecular mechanisms; (3) changes in brain development; and (4) a neurocomputational level. In discussing various disorders, we will briefly review what is known about these other levels of analysis and how that knowledge informs and constrains the neuropsychological explanation of the disorder.

PART II

WHAT ARE THE DISORDERS?

CHAPTER 6

■■■■■■■

Disorders of Perception

T his and the following chapters in this section on disorders will have a common outline that includes (1) *definition*; (2) *brain mechanisms*; (3) *typical development*; and (4) *disorders*. Each chapter will emphasize continuities between normal and abnormal behavior.

DEFINITION

To paraphrase William James, we all know what perception is. Or at least we think we do. The sight of a red rose, the smell of orange blossoms, the taste of chocolate, the caress of a spring breeze on our skin, and the sound of a Beethoven symphony are all products of perception. We experience them as directly given, immediate, and phenomenally real. Such experiences are an important part of what we mean by consciousness and a perennial problem in philosophy, which labels them as qualia, qualitative experiences in contrast to quantitative calculations. If the mind is some kind of computing machine, how can it have vivid, first-person perceptual experiences—that is, qualia?

One of the dramatic surprises for most beginning students of psychology is to find out that the eye is not a sort of camera nor is the ear some kind of telephone. Even neurologists have fallen into this conceptual error. Henschen called area V1, the primary visual cortex, the "cortical retina." Because of our phenomenal experience of *qualia*, we think our sense organs passively deliver a veridical copy of the world. But if that is true, to whom is this copy delivered? Is there a little man sitting in the "Cartesian theatre" (Dennett, 1987) watching a movie of the world? On reflection, of course not, because the little man is a homunculus and we have already discussed the fatal flaw in homuncular explanations. They just push the problem of explanation back one step, so that now we have to explain how perception happens in the head of the little man, and so on. So, as is typically the case in science, we cannot trust the evidence our senses provide, even about our own senses! Our phenomenal experience of perception is deeply misleading about its actual mechanisms (see Metzinger, 2003).

Perception is divided into three broad categories: exteroception, proprioception, and interoception. Exteroception involves perception of the external world, proprioception involves perception of one's own body position and movement, and interoception involves perception of internal states like hunger and thirst. All three kinds of perception produce conscious experience, and the last, interoception, is an aspect of self-consciousness that is not available to an outside observer. All exteroception begins with a **distal object** in the real world, which the brain reconstructs into a representation that is *relevant* for that particular organism. All perception begins with a physical stimulus (materialism again) that receptors in the organism's sense organs can detect.

BRAIN MECHANISMS

So the first structures needed for perception are receptors specialized for different physical stimuli. Most receptors are proteins that are folded in such a way that they can react to the presence of these physical stimuli. Chemoreceptors in the nose and tongue actually bind the molecules from the distal object. Photoreceptors (in rods and cones in the eye) bind to photons to detect wavelengths of light reflected from the distal object, but only the wavelengths relevant for that organism. Thermoceptors are proteins that detect temperature. Nocioceptors are proteins that detect noxious stimuli. Mechanoreceptors, which detect pressure and vibration, work somewhat differently, but still rely on signaling channels, which are proteins. Mechanoreceptors are important in both the sense of touch and hearing. For instance, the hair cells in the inner ear detect pressure changes caused by sound waves. All these various kinds of receptors *transduce* the physical stimulus into a neuronal signal. Importantly, even this transduction is not passive or transparent, but rather selective, as we will explain for the retina of the eye. The pattern of neuronal activity generated by the sense organs is called the proximal stimulus, which is then transmitted to the thalamus, which performs additional processing, and then to primary and secondary and association areas in the cortex, which reconstruct the distal object as a percept or mental representation. (The neural pathways are different for some aspects of interoception like thirst and hunger, which also involve specialized receptors in the periphery, but which project to the hypothalamus.) So, this is a sketch of how the distal object gets "into our head." Later we will discuss how percepts are constructed, which occurs mostly in the neocortex.

Parenthetically, some simple disorders of behavior can be traced to faulty sensory receptors, due to effects in single genes that code for the relevant receptor protein or signaling channel. Congenital blindness and deafness are sometimes caused this way, and everyone is familiar with color blindness, which is due to single gene mutations that affect the retinal cone cells. There are also informative, rarer examples of disorders of behavior caused by faulty sensory receptors. For instance, there are two inherited forms of **achromotopsia** (complete lack of color vision, but also diminished visual acuity and photophobia) that are *channelopathies* (diseases due to a deficient ion channel). One form of peripheral achromotopsia is due to mutations in the gene CNGA3 and the other in CNGB3. Each of these genes codes for subunits of retinal ion channels (Nestler, Hyman, & Malenka, 2009). There are also channelopathies that selectively affect nocioceptors. One example is a rare, recessive single-gene disorder found in three intermarried families in Pakistan. Affected family members were normal in every way except that they could not experience pain, and consequently had lip and tongue injuries from biting themselves as well as bruises and cuts in other places (Nestler et al., 2009). Their mutation was in the SCN9A gene, which forms a component of a particular ion channel (sodium, Na+) that is densely expressed in nociceptive neurons.

Some of these peripheral receptor disorders are a good example of the **subtraction model** for explaining an abnormal behavior, in which one component of behavior is eliminated, leaving all others intact. As we will see, these disorders also make the point that the subtraction model works better for disorders in perception whose cause lies at the sensory surface and not in higher brain centers. For instance, cortical achromotopsia after acquired brain damage is not as specific as sometimes claimed (Zeki, 1992), and affected patients have some preserved color processing and frequent comorbid object agnosias, such as prosopagnosia (Cowey & Heywood, 1997).

Contrary to our phenomenology, our perceptual experiences are filtered and constructed, beginning with our peripheral sense organs. Even though the eye does have a lens, like a camera, the retina is not like film because it is already processing the input. Briefly, the three-layered retina performs contrast enhancement computations that capture how the visual signal changes over space and time. As a consequence, edges of objects are more important to the retina than their homogeneous interior. Scientists have constructed artificial retinas. The output of such an artificial retina is strikingly different from what we perceive using the entire visual system. The retinal output consists of a gray-scale image (no color) with marked, ridge-like edges and no internal detail. It is like a high-contrast filtered image of the object. Viewing the output of an artificial retina is a good way to dispel your naive belief that the eye is a camera. Also unlike a camera, the retina has a different distribution of photoreceptors in the center, or fovea, of the visual field versus the periphery, or parafovea. Cones are densely packed in the fovea, whereas rods are more frequent in the parafovea. The rods are sensitive to low light and movement but are not good at coding visual detail. So, two kinds of visual information are already segregated at the level of the retina. This separation is maintained in the thalamus and the neocortex, the latter of which has a separate visual pathway for "what" information versus "where" or "how" information.

Let us now trace what becomes of the proximal stimulus once it leaves the sensory surface. In the visual system, as discussed above, there are two streams of visual information leaving the retina, one foveal and one parafoveal, both of which project to the lateral geniculate nucleus (LGN) of the thalamus. There is also a parafoveal projection to the superior colliculus in the midbrain, which mediates rapid visual orienting to a peripheral stimulus. Within the six layers of the LGN of the thalamus, the separation of the foveal and parafoveal paths are maintained, with the parafoveal path making connections onto magnocellular neurons in layers 1 and 2, whereas the foveal path connects to parvocellular neurons in layers 3–6. The inputs to the LGN exhibit a general principle of input across most sensory systems, namely **homotopy**, which means that they map the external world in a one-to-one fashion. A dramatic example of homotopy is found in the barrel fields in a rodent's somatosensory cortex (see Figure 6.1), which faithfully map the location of each whisker on the rodent's face (hence, *somotopy*). In the visual system, the homotopy that is found is called **retinotopic**, meaning that the spatial map of the external world projected onto the retina is maintained at the level of the thalamus and at the level of V1 (Brodmann's area 17) in the neocortex. So this kind of analog coding preserves spatial information about visual input without having to code it separately. As a consequence of retinotopy, the visual system divides the world into visual fields, with each eye having a right and left visual field (see Figure 6.2). Normally both eyes converge on a focal point in external space, so that the right and left visual fields in each eye receive similar information, which is only completely in register

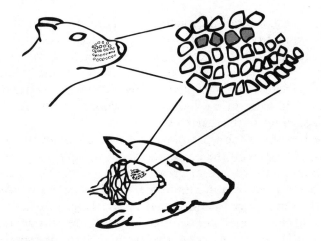

FIGURE 6.1. Homotopy in rodent somatosensory cortex.

for each field in the plane of the focal point. For other planes, either those beyond or before the focal point, the images in each field are slightly out of register, and the brain uses this disparity of information to compute depth information in the visual world (**stereopsis**), as discussed earlier in Chapter 5. Retinotopy requires that the mapping of each visual field is also preserved at the level of the thalamus and neocortex, with the right visual field projections from each eye going to the LGN in the left hemisphere and those from the left visual field going to the LGN in the right hemisphere.

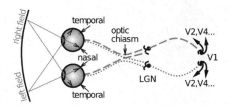

FIGURE 6.2. The pathway of early visual processing from the retina through the lateral geniculate nucleus of the thalamus (LGN) to primary visual cortex (V1), showing how information from the different visual fields (left vs. right) is routed to the opposite hemisphere. From O'Reilly, Munakata, Frank, Hazy, & Contributors (2012). Copyright 2012 by R. C. O'Reilly and Y. Munakata. Reprinted by permission.

Interestingly, most of the inputs to the LGN are downward or feedback projections from V1, outnumbering the feedforward connections from the retina. So, the neocortex, in effect, is telling the LGN which input to prioritize. We only wish our cameras could do that. Similar organizational principles apply to other sensory pathways: homotopy, what versus where (at least, in the auditory system), and feedback projections from the neocortex to the thalamus.

In the neocortex, the separation of foveal and parafoveal information is also maintained, with the parvocellular (foveal) projections synapsing in layers 2 and 3 of V1 and magnocellular (parafoveal) projections synapsing in layer 4. As seen in Figure 6.3, which depicts a monkey brain, from V1 there are projections to secondary visual areas: first to V2 (which has thick and thin stripes, not depicted in the figure, that are devoted to parafoveal and foveal inputs, respectively) and then to areas specialized for dynamic form (V3), and color and form with color (V4). Area V4 is part of the **ventral visual pathway**, which specializes in *what* information and projects forward into inferior temporal areas that are specialized for visual object representations. Area V3 is part of the **dorsal visual pathway**, which specializes in *where* or *how* information, and they project forward to parts of the parietal lobe that code spatial reference frames important

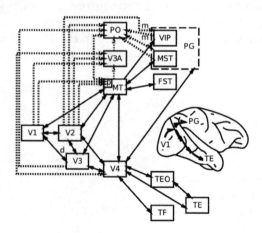

FIGURE 6.3. Division of "what" versus "where" (ventral vs. dorsal) visual pathways in a monkey brain. Solid lines are full visual field projections, while dotted lines are peripheral visual field. From O'Reilly, Munakata, Frank, Hazy, and Contributors (2012). Copyright 2012 by R. C. O'Reilly and Y. Munakata. Reprinted by permission.

for both localizing objects in space and planning bodily movements (so, the dorsal path is also called the *"how"* pathway).

Moving further along the ventral visual stream into the inferior temporal (IT) cortex, one encounters neurons that are increasingly specific in the visual stimuli they respond to. Such cells are called "grandmother cells" (by critics) and are often said to be uniquely responsive to highly complex stimuli, such as an individual face. This extreme localization of function, first criticized by Lashley in the quote at the beginning of Chapter 3 (Lashley & Clark, 1946) is improbable for both logical and empirical reasons. Given the seemingly unlimited capacity of visual cortex to learn to recognize new objects, there may not be enough neurons in the IT to code for each individual object. Also, such a system would be very vulnerable to damage; what if the grandmother neuron died? Instead, we now know that visual object recognition and many other aspects of brain function are remarkably robust and exhibit graceful (instead of abrupt) degradation in the face of damage. A single percept is not abruptly lost after damage, and damage does not selectively damage just one percept. Another problem with such a sparse or localist coding system is that it would exhibit limited generalizability, a key problem that doomed S-R accounts of behavior. We recognize not just our grandmother, but caricatures of Grandmother, Grandmother at different ages, women who look like our grandmother, and so on. To empirically test the grandmother cell theory, we need to sample many adjacent IT cells and test whether multiple cells contribute to coding a specific object as opposed to just one. When this has been done, the results indeed support population coding of visual objects (see Banich & Compton, 2011). Population coding is an example of vector coding, discussed earlier. In population coding, the representation of a particular face is distributed over a population of neurons, which are also involved in the coding of other faces. Each individual face is thus a point in a multivariate face space, and faces that are closer in face space are perceived as more similar. Such a coding arrangement permits the extraction of more abstract dimensions of faces, such as gender, age, ethnicity, and emotion, as well as the recognition of caricatures.

Population coding is also consistent with other well-known properties of perception, such as perceptual constancy and its categorical nature. Perceptual constancy means that same object is recognized regardless of size, orientation, shading and color, and even some degree of occlusion or masking. Categorical perception means that exemplars of a given object (e.g., a rabbit) that share features of another perceptual object (e.g., a duck) are still perceived as belonging to one category or another, not as a hybrid. Categorical perception is demonstrated empirically by morphing one object into another in a series of small steps and then presenting each image individually for a recognition judgment. If subjects' perception was continuous, their rate of identifying each image as one object (e.g., rabbit) would gradually decline as the image became more like the other object (e.g., a duck). Instead, their recognition rates for one object are similar until the category boundary is reached and then abruptly switch to high recognition rates for the other object. So, instead of being linear, the recognition function approximates a threshold or sigmoid function. We will find these aspects of perception again in Chapter 8 when we discuss speech perception and show how it is similar in important ways to visual object perception.

Perceptual constancy and categorical perception make it clear that recognition of a perceptual object is an active, integrative process. The integrative or constructive aspect of perception is dramatically illustrated by perceptual illusions. In the domain of visual perception, two of the earliest illusions to be described and studied are the Necker illusion (Figure 6.4) and the Müller–Lyer illusion (Figure 6.5). The Necker illusion is usually presented as a cube, but Necker initially presented it as a rhomboid, which is shown in Figure 6.4. The Necker illusion has two aspects: (1) we infer depth from a two-dimensional drawing (why not just see it as a flat pattern of tiles?) and (2) our perception alternates (i.e., perceptual rivalry) between a rhomboid that protrudes out and one that protrudes in. In the Müller–Lyer illusion (Figure 6.5), we are asked to compare the length of two horizontal line segments of equal length, and we judge them as having different lengths. This illusion arises because our perceptual processing integrates *all* the visual cues in the figure, the task-irrelevant small

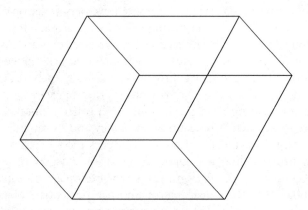

FIGURE 6.4. Necker illusion.

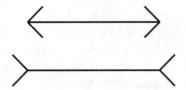

FIGURE 6.5. Müller–Lyer illusion.

diagonal lines that resemble the point or feathers of an arrow, and the two horizontal lines we are asked to judge.

TYPICAL DEVELOPMENT

Endogenous neural activity and then environmental stimulation are necessary for sensory and perceptual systems to develop properly, and primary sensory areas in the neocortex are plastic and can function for other sensory modalities if they are experimentally rewired or deprived of their ordinary inputs (as in congenital deafness or blindness). Because many of the synapses involved in sensation and perception are formed after birth and remodeled across the life span in an experience-dependent fashion, it is essentially impossible for there to be innate circuits for many percepts like human faces or phonemes (see Elman et al., 1996; Greenough et al., 1987; E. P. Johnson, Pennington, Lowenstein, & Nittrover, 2011). Nonetheless, some aspects of sensation and perception are developing in an experience-dependent fashion *before* birth, based on sensory stimuli that can reach the fetus. For hearing, we know that sensation and perception begin to develop before birth because neonates can distinguish their mother's voice. Further, taste preferences are influenced by the mother's diet during pregnancy, and the infant's stress-response system is being affected by the pregnant mother's experience. The latter two cases are examples of "fetal programming," a burgeoning new field in developmental psychology. Obviously, the fetus gets very limited visual input, and postnatal visual development lags behind auditory development, yet infants in the first week of life are able to identify their mother visually based on the general shape of her head and hair, although not on the configuration of facial features (Pascalis, de Schonen, Morton, Deruelle, & Fabre-Grenet, 1995).

As will be discussed below, although infants may have an innate bias for orienting to face-like stimuli, facial recognition skills develop in a way that is consistent with interactive specialization theory discussed earlier. Only a few decades ago, neonates were assumed to be blind. Marshall Haith (1966) and other developmental psychologists proved that this was not the case. Postnatal perceptual development proceeds consistent with the general principle of interactive specialization, explained earlier (see also Glossary). Babies learn the species-typical perceptual invariances in an experience expectant way, as explained in Chapter 5. They overproduce synapses in the sensory and perceptual circuits and then prune those based on nearly universal sensory inputs. As also discussed in Chapter 5, this is how ocular dominance columns are formed in V1 early in postnatal life, with each column being specific to input from a single eye. Also as discussed earlier, binocular visual experience is necessary for the ocular dominance columns to form, and deprivation of such input during the critical period leads to permanent visual defects, notably a failure of stereoscopic vision.

Percepts that are more culturally or individual specific (a particular language or particular faces) are learned more slowly in an experience-dependent way, with new synapses being created and nonfunctional ones being pruned away, as explained in Chapter 5. Children's visual object perception reaches an adult level in many ways by preschool age, but speech perception has a more protracted course, as we will discuss later in Chapter 8, on language disorders.

DISORDERS

Damage to the brain can produce sensory deficits in a given modality. For instance, bilateral destruction of V1 produces cortical blindness and bilateral destruction of Heschl's gyrus (A1) produces cortical deafness. Certain neurological disorders, such as a closed head injury, can damage the primary olfactory and gustatory cortex in the orbitofrontal cortex and result in a loss of the senses of smell and taste. Unilateral damage to primary somatosensory cortex produces lack of tactile and proprioceptive sensation on the contralateral side of the body: when touched on that side (while blindfolded), the patient reports nothing. All of these examples look like straightforward examples of the **subtraction model** for explaining an abnormal behavior: damage to a certain brain region is necessary and sufficient to eliminate a function. Are they really that simple? We now know that they are not, based on work by Weiskrantz (1986) and Zeki (1992) on cortical blindness. Patients with cortical blindness can identify the location of visual stimuli above chance level, all the while denying that they see anything. This surprising condition is called **blindsight**, and it demonstrates that visual awareness (an aspect of consciousness) is partly dissociable from low-level visual detection. One explanation of blindsight is that subcortical visual pathways (i.e., those in the superior colliculus) are still intact and still connected to brain areas that support a voluntary motor response, pointing.

Perception and recognition can be disrupted by lesions to secondary areas for the various sensory modalities, and these can occur for higher and lower levels of processing. Consistent with a classical localization of function approach, some 20th-century vision researchers (e.g., Zeki, 1992) have emphasized "pure" cases that appear to damage a single visual function. As discussed earlier, some patients with damage to V4 (the color and form area in the occipital cortex) lose color vision, a condition called cortical achromotopsia, but they have other problems with visual perception as well. Zeki (1992) also describes a syndrome called **chromotopsia**—apparently the opposite of achromotopsia—in which color vision is preserved but form vision is lost. Zeki (1992) uses this apparent double dissociation to argue that color and form perception are independent localized functions. But the fact that these cases are rarely pure and the problems with double dissociation logic discussed in Chapter 3 both call into question this conclusion. A third such syndrome is **akinetopsia**, in which area V5 is damaged and perception of motion is disrupted.

The disorders that are most informative about visual perception are visual agnosias. The term **agnosia** was coined by Sigmund Freud, who was a neurologist by training, and means "without knowledge." (You have probably noticed by now that many neurological syndromes begin with the prefix *a*- which means "without.") So, the problem in agnosia is not in sensation, but in perception and recognition. The classical classification of visual agnosias, going back to Lissauer in the 1890s, distinguishes **apperceptive** from **associative** agnosia, with the former being a problem in perception of visual objects and the latter being a problem of associating the visual percept of an object with its meaning, resulting in impaired recognition of visual objects by patients with visual associative agnosia. So, these two types of visual agnosia implied a potential double dissociation in which perception of and memory for visual objects (permitting recognition) are independent stages of processing. On testing, apperceptive agnosics cannot copy visually presented objects, although their processing of component visual features like lines or angles appears intact. This deficit in copying visual objects would be consistent with a deficit in perception, which requires that elementary features like lines and angles be integrated into a global whole. If perception is prior to and necessary for recognition, then apperceptive agnosics will also fail to recognize visual objects, but not because their memory of visual objects is impaired.

In contrast, associative agnosics can produce good drawings of a visually presented object, implying intact perception, but cannot say what the object is (a failure of recognition), implying a selective deficit in accessing memory for visual objects, either because of disconnection or because the memory representations themselves are damaged. Both types of agnosics can name the same objects through feeling them with their hands and describe the object's function, so they have some intact semantic memory for the objects they cannot perceive visually and do not have a name retrieval problem. Consequently, the neuropsychological explanation of associative agnosia is somewhat puzzling, because object recognition is not totally missing, just when objects are presented visually. These two types of visual agnosia are associated with different brain lesions: diffuse bilateral occipital lobe lesions in the case of apperceptive agnosia and more localized bilateral damage at the occipitotemporal border in associative agnosia, consistent with a later stage of visual processing.

However, the dissociation between the two types of agnosia is not as clearcut as the classical accounts imply. More recent studies have found subtle perceptual problems in associative agnosics. For instance, their good drawings of visual objects are accomplished in a detail-by-detail, piecemeal fashion, instead of by drawing the global form and adding details as typical controls do. Moreover, no cases of a pure recognition problem in associative agnosia have been found (Farah, 2003), so the dissociation between perception and memory for visual objects is not complete. Connectionist models in which the same units are used in both perception and memory for visual objects have been used to simulate both types of visual agnosia. So, once again we have an example where a focus on seeming pure cases and box-and-arrow models of processing have been misleading about the actual brain mechanisms underlying a disorder, in this case visual agnosia. The connectionist account is more parsimonious because it does not have separate components for perception and memory and more consistent with the empirical evidence from agnosics, as well as with separate evidence from neuroimaging studies that demonstrate that the same brain posterior regions mediate visual perception and visual imagery (which depends on memory representations of visual objects).

Is Face Recognition a Module?

There are somewhat more specific examples of visual agnosia, the most studied being **prosopagnosia**, an inability to recognize faces, either because of an acquired lesion or due to a developmental disorder (i.e., congenital prosopagnosia). Research on typical and disordered face perception has been a major focus in cognitive neuroscience over the last 10 years or so, and the debate over whether face recognition is an evolved human module (see discussion of Fodor's [1983] modularity theory in Chapter 3) has been intense and continues. Before stepping into the evidence and the debate, it is useful to cite some lessons from debates about innate modules for syntax, phonology, and theory of mind, which are discussed in more detail later in this book. In these cases, it was argued that because there were inherited disorders in each domain (language impairment [LI], dyslexia, and autism, respectively) there might be genes for coding for each module. Similar to our light switch example discussed earlier and to the arguments in Chapter 3 on localization of brain function, we can say quite clearly that the localization of a gene or genes that disrupt the development of a given function is not the localization of all the genes involved in that function. Second, in each of these cases, it became clear that the behavioral deficits in the disorder involved were broader than assumed. Third, it was found that learning and development are important in each of these syndromes, and the same is likely to be true in developmental prosopagnosia.

The modular position in this debate about the brain basis of face recognition is that humans have an evolved, innate face recognition area, located in the fusiform gyrus of the ventral occipitotemporal cortex (the fusiform face area [FFA]). So, this FFA would meet Fodor's (1983) definition of a cognitive module and would be consistent with a maturational theory of development. One highly respected advocate of this position is Nancy Kanwisher (e.g., 2010). In this publication, she reviews the evidence and arguments for regarding the FFA as a module. There are two main competitors to the modular, maturational theory of the FFA. One is the interactive specialization theory proposed by Johnson and de Haan (2011) and briefly discussed earlier in Chapter 4. The other is the skill-learning theory proposed by Gauthier and Nelson (2001). Both of these theories agree that learning is critical to acquiring the skill of face recognition and that brain–behavior relations develop. The key difference between these two theories is whether localization of functions changes with development. In interactive specialization, interactions among connected brain areas in development will change the localization of a function, often by shrinking it as expertise accumulates (e.g., the whole neocortex is active in language acquisition in infancy, but eventually the function of language becomes largely lateralized to the left hemisphere). In the skill-learning theory, the same brain substrates are important for a given function in both infants and adults. Moreover, skill learning assumes the greatest plasticity in brain development of the three theories: maturational, interactive specialization, and skill learning.

We can roughly map these three theories onto the epistemological theories discussed in Chapter 2. Skill theory roughly corresponds to empiricism: knowledge comes from the environment and is not innate. In contrast, the maturational or modular theory corresponds roughly to idealism and its instantiation in certain forms of evolutionary psychology: knowledge acquisition depends on innate, specialized modules that evolved. Interactive specialization is an intermediate position between these two extremes and corresponds to Piagetian constructivism. Piaget developed his constructivist theory to address the nature versus nurture debate regarding the question of where ideas or knowledge come from. Constructivism holds that there are innate constraints on how knowledge can be acquired and what knowledge is important, but it is the interaction of those constraints with experience that leads to the development of knowledge.

All three theories agree that the particular inputs and outputs of a given brain region, which develop before birth, limit the eventual function of that specific brain region. So, based on their input/output wiring, only certain brain regions could become specialized for visual object recognition (e.g., not secondary olfactory, auditory, or somatosensory cortex). But the three positions disagree on whether there are innate **content constraints** on connectivity-determined candidate neural substrates for visual object recognition. The maturational theory holds that the FFA is innately dedicated to faces as its preferred content. Interactive specialization holds that there is innate, subcortically mediated orienting bias for even very minimal face-like stimuli (e.g., a triangular array of three dots within a circle) that guarantees human infants will spend a lot of time looking at faces. But interactive specialization holds that the content specialization of the FFA will emerge over time and that other additional structures besides the fusiform gyrus will participate in face perception earlier in development. Skill-learning theory posits that the entire fusiform area is a good candidate substrate for visual object recognition, but that different fusiform subregions develop expertise for given contents because of extensive practice and the timing of the environmental input. So, skill theory holds that different learning histories would lead to different specializations in the same brain region for other contents. On this view, the FFA is a face area just because humans typically practice recognition of human faces more and earlier than they practice recognition of any other object (e.g., animal faces, cars, visual words). Consequently, different learning histories could produce different content specializations in the FFA.

Finally, all three theories agree that recognition of *particular* faces develops (i.e., it cannot be innate) and continues for an individual's entire life, barring brain damage or dementia. The whole point of our ability to rapidly learn individual facial identities and discriminate thousands of different faces is to deal with the many individual people we encounter in our lives. So, learning about individual faces is an example of experience-dependent synaptogenesis, which continues throughout the life span. We can keep learning about new faces as we age, just as we can keep learning new words. Thus, the innate content specialization of the FFA must be about a particular cognitive process that is unique to face recognition, such as configural processing. Now that we have explained the three competing theories, let us turn to the relevant evidence.

Ironically, most of the research on the brain bases of face recognition has been done in adults, even though the crucial evidence for deciding between the theories depends on how adult competence develops. This disproportionate emphasis on adults is more for practical and historical reasons than substantive ones, and is true in all domains of human neuroscience covered in this book. On the practical side, it is easier to do research on adults than children. Historically, there have been many more graduate training programs in adult cognitive neuroscience than in developmental cognitive neuroscience.

Neuroscience research on face recognition in adults has yielded some findings that all three theoretical positions would predict and other findings that distinguish them. In the first category of shared predicted findings we have the following:

1. Adult face perception, more than other forms of object recognition, is particularly dependent on configural processing. Configural processing is indexed behaviorally by the **inversion effect**, meaning that adults have considerably more difficulty recognizing an inverted face than an upright face. The inversion effect is not found with non-face objects (Yin, 1970).
2. Face processing in adults has a specific neuroimaging signature both in fMRI studies (i.e., selection activation of the FFA) and in ERP studies (i.e., the N170). These signatures of face processing are somewhat lateralized to the right hemisphere, consistent with the known specialization of the right hemisphere for configural processing (see reviews in Banich & Compton, 2011; Gazzaniga, Ivry, & Magnun, 2009).
3. There are persons with acquired prosopagnosia who have relatively specific deficits in the recognition of human faces (Farah, 1994). So all three theories agree that adults have specialized and

localized processing of human faces that can be damaged selectively.

Which adult findings distinguish these three competing theories? Studies of expertise by Gauthier and colleagues have shown that car and bird experts activate the FFA in an fMRI study in which they had to discriminate particular cars and birds (Gauthier, Skudlarski, Gore, & Anderson, 2000). Moreover, Gauthier, Tarr, Anderson, Skudlarski, and Gore (1999) found that intense training to discriminate the "faces" of invented creatures (eyeless, bird-like heads with varying beaks and crowns, called "Greebles") leads to right FFA activation for Greeble experts, who also begin to show an inversion effect (Gauthier et al., 1999). These findings challenge the notion that the human FFA is a module strictly specialized for a specific content and instead show that it exhibits considerable plasticity.

In acquired prosopagnosia, sometimes expertise for other within-class object discriminations is lost, as in the case of a farmer who lost the ability to recognize individual cows in his herd or a bird-watcher who lost the ability to individuate birds in a given species. But in other cases of acquired prosopagnosia, the two abilities dissociate, as was found in a car expert who retained his car recognition ability or a sheep farmer who retained his ability to recognize individual sheep (see review in Banich & Compton, 2011). But it is hard to see how these four case studies are decisive for either the modular or the skill-learning theory. All they demonstrate is that face expertise sometimes dissociates from other within-class expertise and sometimes not, which is not surprising given the variability both in acquired lesions and an individual's brain specializations. The dissociation between face and other within-class expertise would only pose a difficulty for the skill-learning theory if it were postulating that there is only *one* expertise area in the brain, which it is not.

Two other findings pose considerable challenges for the modular theory of the FFA. One is that there appear to be nonface clusters of neurons within the FFA, based on a study that used high-resolution fMRI (Grill-Spector, Sayres, & Ress, 2006). The other is a study by Haxby et al. (2001) that used a novel, synthetic method to examine the function of the FFA and adjacent brain regions. The typical approach to defining the FFA in fMRI studies is to select those voxels that are significantly more activated by faces than by control stimuli. Since that selection depends on a statistical cutoff imposed on continuous data, some of the nonselected voxels are activated by faces, just not as much as the selected ones. Likewise, the selected voxels that are deemed face-selective can be activated by other stimuli besides faces. The key question addressed by the Haxby et al. (2001) study was whether the activity of the nonselected voxels could perform the behavioral task of face recognition. To answer this question, they dropped the face-selective voxels from the data set and used only the activity levels of the nonselected voxels. The activity of these nonselected voxels was the input to a multivariate pattern-classifying algorithm whose task was to perform the facial discrimination task subjects had performed in the scanner. The surprising and important result was that nonselected voxels were nearly as accurate as the face-selective ones. These results are consistent with distributed population coding of face and other object representations in the FFA and its neighbors (see also Hanson & Halchenko, 2008). They argue against highly specialized, sparse, or localist coding.

Kanwisher (2010) discusses both these results, which pose a challenge for her modular theory. She claims that a module does not have to be a single "island" in the brain but can be an archipelago to deal with the Grill-Spector et al. (2006) results. She concedes the Haxby et al. (2001) result that nonselective voxels contain information about faces but argues that they are not important in real-world face processing and are more of an epiphenomenon.

So, the adult literature does not seem absolutely conclusive for the two competing theories (modularity and skill theory), and different reviews have come to different conclusions about whether either theory is favored by the evidence and which one. My own opinion is that the expertise studies by Gautier and colleagues and the research by Grill-Spector et al. (2006) and Haxby et al. (2001) tip the balance toward the skill theory, but other experts would certainly disagree. So, let us turn to the more crucial developmental evidence.

The modular theory is supported by *some* evidence that face processing does not develop slowly in childhood, as was previously thought (e.g., Carey & Diamond, 1977), and that key behavioral markers of adult-like face processing are present in some studies as early as age 3 and even earlier in others (McKone, Crookes, Jeffery, & Dilks, 2012), but are not observed until adolescence in some studies (Golarai et al., 2007; Scherf, Behrmann, Humphreys, & Luna, 2007). However, even if face processing develops faster than previously thought, it is certainly not fully present at birth. Infants become better at processing faces with experience, and they develop gender and race facial preferences consistent with that experience (Ramsey-Rennels & Langlois, 2006).

Other reviews of the development of face processing, especially in infancy, provide strong evidence for both the skill-learning and interactive specialization theories (Gauthier & Nelson, 2001; Johnson & de Haan, 2011) and against the modular, maturational theory. Probably the most telling finding is that the use of configural processing of faces is not present at birth, and develops slowly over the first year of life, and requires visual experience. As discussed earlier, an innate special processing mechanism is at the heart of the modular theory, and the inversion effect is the key behavioral marker of configural processing. Studies in the first year of life indicate that preferential processing of upright faces is *not* present at birth, and that facial inversion only makes a difference in infant behavioral performance at 5 months (Bhatt, Bertin, Hayden, & Reed, 2005). The inversion effect becomes apparent in the N170 evoked response on an EEG at 12 months, although an N170 response to faces is detectable by 3 months (Johnson & de Haan, 2011). Visual disruption by infantile cataracts prevents the development of configural processing of faces, indicating that experience is necessary (Mondloch, Le Grand, & Maurer, 2003), even though the cataracts are removed later. Neuroimaging studies of the FFA in children are consistent with the predictions of the interactive specialization theory in that face processing becomes localized with development. For instance Scherf et al. (2007) found the FFA specialization for faces was not present in children as old as 5–8 years, because the FFA was equally activated by objects and landscapes, whereas occipital object areas and the parahippocampal place area did exhibit specialization by that age.

An additional piece of developmental evidence to consider comes from developmental prosopagnosia, in which explicit facial recognition deficits can be impressively selective. Nonetheless, people with this disorder are not missing an FFA, as an extreme modularity theory would predict, and their FFA is activated by faces, but not as specifically as those of typical individuals (Duchaine & Nakayama, 2006). As with a syndrome like blindsight, implicit processing of facial identity by persons with prosopagnosia is above chance levels (Avidan & Behrmann, 2008; Eimer, Gosling, & Duchaine, 2012; Rivolta, Palermo, Schmalzl, & Coltheart, 2012; Rivolta, Schmalzl, Coltheart, & Palermo, 2011), and they have an electrodermal response to familiar faces despite not recognizing them. Training can improve their deficit somewhat, increasing the face selectivity of their N170 ERP (DeGutis & D'Esposito, 2007). Eimer et al. (2012) interpret these results in developmental prosopagnosia as being consistent with a **disconnection** explanation of the deficit in which visual face recognition units in the brain are not communicating with downstream semantic brain areas representing personal identity.

Another perspective on this theoretical debate is provided by the role of the fusiform word area, also called the visual word form area (VWFA), which is anatomically close to the FFA. The VWFA slowly becomes specialized for printed word recognition in childhood over several years of reading experience, and this specialization is less developed in children with dyslexia. But since reading is a cultural invention, no one is arguing for an innate evolved reading module in the VWFA. In addition to their anatomical similarity, there are several other similarities between developmental prosopagnosia and developmental dyslexia. Both are fairly specific, genetically influenced deficits in processing particular visual objects (faces or words). Both appear to involve disconnection, although much more is known about the disruptions in white matter connectivity in dyslexia. Both respond, at least partially, to remediation. Because of these similarities, it is more parsimonious to propose similar developmental mechanisms for both disorders. Another piece of evidence supporting this conclusion is provided by a third disorder, autism.

Problems in face recognition occur in autism, another genetically influenced neurodevelopmental disorder, but apparently for experiential reasons (see Schultz, 2005, for a review). Because individuals with autism do not orient to faces or people and exhibit different eye movement patterns when they do look at faces, they are not getting the extensive practice with faces that typical children do. Individuals with autism do not activate the FFA in face recognition tasks, providing additional evidence that experience is important for the development of the specialization of the FFA for faces. A counterargument could be that people with autism have congenital problems with the FFA, namely that the cause of their autism is developmental prosopagnosia. But the fact that most individuals with developmental prosopagnosia do not have autism argues strongly against the hypothesis that congenital prosopagnosia is sufficient to cause autism.

CHAPTER SUMMARY

An important aspect of our conscious experience, the perception of visual objects, develops in both an experience-expectant and experience-dependent way. Visual representations used in the recognition of familiar objects must be sufficiently abstract to permit perceptual invariance, and these abstract representations are mediated by populations of neurons in the ventral visual stream. Although specializations for different classes of objects (faces, printed words, places, etc.) can develop, these specializations do not appear to be absolute or innately determined modules, and are better accounted for by the skill-learning or interactive specialization theories.

EXERCISES

1. What exactly is stereoscopic vision? If you have trouble seeing the three-dimensional images in "magic" stereogram pictures, you may be concerned you don't have it. However, if you've gotten this far in life, chances are you see stereoscopically like the majority of humans. To test it, sit facing a wall or distant object, about 15 feet from that object. Hold up your pen in front of your face and look past the pen to the object on the wall—how many pens do you now see? If you answered two, then congratulations! You have stereoscopic vision. Your eyes are actually each processing the image of this pen separately. Now refocus on the pen; the two images should merge back to one, demonstrating how your cortex makes sense of the two images projected on each of your retinas. Bonus: Which group of humans do *not* have stereoscopic vision, and why?

2. Search for "blindsight" on YouTube and you will likely come up with many videos on this disorder. I like Ramachandran's segment about what blindsight reveals about consciousness. If that isn't available, however, look for a video that demonstrates one of the "unconscious" motor reactions of blindsight patients to visual objects, despite their lack of visual awareness. Bonus: How do we know these patients are not faking their lack of conscious sight?

CHAPTER 7

Disorders of Attention

Everyone knows what attention is. It is the taking possession by the mind, in clear and vivid form, of one out of what seem several simultaneously possible objects or trains of thought. Focalization, concentration of consciousness are of its essence. It implies withdrawal from some things in order to deal effectively with others, and is a condition which has a real opposite in the confused, dazed, scatterbrain state.

—JAMES (1890, p. 403)

DEFINITION

Most psychologists have read James's definition of attention before, some with the wry reaction that we still do not really know what attention is more than 100 years later. But James's definition captures several aspects of attention that modern cognitive neuroscientists would agree are crucial: (1) attention is a conscious process; "unconscious attention" is practically an oxymoron, (2) attention has limited capacity and involves both selection and deselection (competition) among a multitude of candidate objects of attention, (3) attention can be effortful and is not usually an automatic process, (4) attention is closely tied to action and goals for action, so that what we focus our attention on is based on its relevance to us—thus different individuals can attend to very different aspects of the same external event, and (5) there is an intimate relation between normal and abnormal attention, and typical people can have lapses of attention (especially when tired, intoxicated, or overaroused emotionally).

Unlike perception, specific examples of which (e.g., face and speech perception) qualify as vertical faculties or modules in Fodor's (1983) influential classification scheme, attention is clearly a horizontal faculty because it is a cognitive process that operates across diverse contents and modalities. We attend or disattend to exteroceptive and proprioceptive senses (smells, tastes, sights, sounds, touch, etc.), interoceptive senses (e.g., pain, thirst, hunger), and emotions. But we also attend or disattend to memories, future goals, and mental imagery. Patients with neglect have deficits in attention that extend across modalities and mental images. Much less research has been done on whether they neglect interoceptive senses and emotions, which are not organized spatially, with pain being an interesting exception (because it is localized to a body part). Fodor (1983) claimed on theoretical grounds that we would forever lack a neuropsychology of horizontal faculties. Thirty years later, it is ironic that we have a very developed cognitive neuroscience of attention and other horizontal faculties like long-term memory and executive functions. If anything, there is less controversy about the neural substrates of these horizontal faculties than about those of the vertical ones (as we saw in the previous chapter's review of the FFA). As we will see in this chapter and later ones, there is also less plasticity for horizontal faculties than vertical ones, because horizontal faculties rely more on convergence zones and specialized neural computations.

BRAIN MECHANISMS

As with the other horizontal faculties, attention is served by a distributed brain network. The brain's visual attention network converges in the parietal cortex and uses a specialized neural computation or representation, namely varying spatial reference frames that the dorsal stream of the extended visual system is specialized for computing. Much of attention is tied to a specific spatial reference frame, and attention can be directed overtly or covertly to various locations in that reference frame. The reference frames can be midline-centered, head-centered, or object-centered. Unlike the ventral visual stream (the "what" system), which conducts many of its operations without consciousness, most operations of the dorsal stream (the "how" system) are intimately tied to consciousness because they involve attention and intention: that is, selection of objects of attention that are relevant to the individual's goals and selection of actions relevant to attain those goals.

Because attention is a conscious process, we can make an important theoretical distinction between perception and attention. Perception can be conscious or unconscious. Some of the processes that construct an object of perception are preattentive, and thus are aspects of unconscious or implicit cognition. Moreover, these same processes are involved in recollection and imagery, so that we may have a mental representation of something recalled or imagined but only attend to part of it. As we will see below, a striking example of this phenomenon is found in representational neglect (Bisiach & Luzzatti, 1978). So, as James's definition makes clear, while perception identifies multiple objects based on the current sensory input, only attention selects which of those objects deserves the coordinated focus of the brain in order to achieve goals of the organism.

Of course, in James's time, little was known about the cognitive and brain mechanisms of attention, and an enormous amount has been learned since then, as we will discuss shortly. Attention is a key topic in cognitive science, but it is relevant to all of psychology. Attention is intimately related to action and emotion regulation and is impaired in different ways in virtually all psychiatric and neurodevelopmental disorders, so that treatment of attention problems is a key issue for clinicians. For instance, in mood and anxiety disorders, there are strong attentional biases toward particular emotional content (sad content in major depression and dysthymia, threatening content in anxiety disorders, particular trauma-related memories in posttraumatic stress disorder (PTSD), and rewarding content in mania and hypomania) that limit the individual's adaptive behavior. These attentional biases and the cognitive distortions to which they lead are a key focus of treatment of these disorders. And of course, impairments of attention are key features of schizophrenia, autism, intellectual disabilities, ADHD, and various learning disorders, each in different ways. When we discuss these disorders, we will explain how attention is disturbed in each.

One key discovery of cognitive science is just how fallible typical adult attention is. We all have attentional "blinks" and can neglect very salient aspects of a scene (e.g., a gorilla walking in front of a group of people) when we are concentrating on other aspects of the scene. So, we literally cannot believe our eyes when it comes to being aware of what is in front of us. For a convincing demonstration of this phenomenon, ask any auto insurance claims adjustor how people explain their accidents (e.g., "A tree jumped out and hit my car"). All of us have auto and other accidents because of lapses in attention that cause us to not see some very relevant thing in front of us. Because of the competitive nature of attention, all of us are susceptible to temporary episodes of attentional neglect and even to **simultagnosia**, the inability to attend to more than one object at a time. We will see that more extreme unbalanced competition helps explain pathological **hemineglect** or hemi-attention, in which patients are unaware of the whole left (or sometimes right) side of the scene or object in front of them, and **Bálint syndrome**, in which there is profound simultagnosia.

An example of simultagnosia in typical humans is provided by the phenomena of perceptual and binocular rivalry. Everyone has seen ambiguous figures, such as the Necker cube or the old versus young woman, in which one's perception of the figure spontaneously shifts without any change in the external stimulus. Such ambiguous figures illustrate **perceptual rivalry**, the inability of the brain to perceive two conflicting interpretations of the input at the same time. Both interpretations are processed implicitly, but attention must select one or the other for conscious experience and a verbal report by the subject. Similarly, in **binocular rivalry**, dissimilar visual inputs are provided to both eyes simultaneously (e.g., one's own left hand in front of the left eye and a vase of flowers viewed through a cardboard tube held in front of the right eye). Instead of our being conscious of both objects, reported visual experience (our conscious attention) alternates between seeing the hand and seeing the flowers. In contrast to pathological simultagnosia, which is discussed later, typical individuals can consciously see two objects at once when using both eyes. But both kinds of simultagnosia, normal and pathological, make the point that attention, unlike preattentive perceptual processing, has a limited capacity and necessarily involves competition, selection, and deselection.

The alternation of conscious attention in perceptual rivalry has been studied with neuroimaging methods in both humans (Lumer, Friston, & Rees, 1998) and monkeys (Logothetis, 1999) with converging results. These are elegant experiments because the phenomenon of perceptual rivalry allows one to isolate neural areas involved only in attentional shifts (when perceptual experience shifts) and distinguish them from neural areas involved in the partly preattentive processing of the visual input, which is constant across shifts in perceptual experience. We would expect the neural areas involved in these attentional shifts to be similar to those identified with other experimental methods (discussed later), and that is indeed the case. In both monkeys and humans, activity in secondary visual areas (i.e., V4 and V5) and in the ventral visual pathway (i.e., inferior temporal cortex) changed with perceptual transitions, whereas activity in V1 changed little in the monkeys (about 10% of recorded neurons) and not at all in humans. Single-unit recordings (the activity of single neurons recorded with microelectrodes) in the monkey study (Logothetis, 1999) were limited to visual areas and the ventral visual pathway, but the human study (Lumer et al., 1998) recorded activity changes in the whole brain and found that distributed right frontoparietal activity was correlated with perceptual transitions. This is the same network that is involved in spatial attention and neglect, as discussed below.

Parenthetically, the monkey study included a manipulation of consciousness. Monkeys were anesthetized and presented with a rotating high-contrast visual stimulus. The visual thalamus (LGN), V1 and secondary visual areas, and medial temporal cortex (MT/V5) were activated by this stimulus, demonstrating that a great deal of visual processing can occur without consciousness. The Logothetis study (1999) also partly addresses the "who has consciousness" problem discussed in Chapter 2: the monkeys were trained when awake to pull a lever when their perceptual experience shifted. Their success with this task is evidence that they are conscious if perceptual rivalry requires consciousness (which it does in humans) and if their lever pulling is accurate. We can infer that it was accurate because it correlated with the objective criterion of changes in single-unit activity in secondary visual areas and inferior temporal cortex also observed in humans. Although one can always claim that the monkeys are unconscious zombies constructed to simulate perceptual rivalry, this argument lacks parsimony, since the monkeys' brain activity was different when they were anesthetized and when they were awake. To accommodate this fact, the zombie argument would have to posit two kinds of unconsciousness in monkeys: one that looks like human unconsciousness and one that looks like human consciousness. As we will see below, work on the development of attention in human infants provides another answer to the "who" question—namely human neonates, who have sleep–wake cycles and exhibit a basic form of conscious attention in the wakeful state.

What else have cognitive scientists and neuroscientists learned about attention in the over 100 years since James's definition? As is the case for most other cognitive processes discussed in this book, cognitive researchers have found evidence for multiple different types of attention with somewhat distinct but interacting neural mechanisms. In the case of attention, three main types have been identified. The most basic level of attention is **alertness and arousal**, the state we are in when we are fully awake, and which we lack when we are in non-rapid-eye-movement (non-REM) sleep, under anesthesia, or in a coma (see Figure 2.1). As discussed earlier, distributed activation of the neocortex is required for a wakeful state or basic consciousness, and this distributed activation has a neuroimaging signature that is measurable with EEG or fMRI. The **reticular activating system (RAS)** controls overall arousal, including regulation of sleep–wake cycles, and consists of the reticular formation and projections to both the hypothalamus (ventral route) and thalamus (dorsal route). Projections from the thalamus stimulate the cortex, whereas sleep-regulating portions of the hypothalamus project back to brainstem nuclei involved in arousal. Three portions of the thalamus are involved in arousal: the medial dorsal, intralaminar, and reticular nuclei. The RAS relies on glutamate, which is the main excitatory neurotransmitter in the brain, to stimulate the structures it projects to and regulate arousal. Parallel cholinergic and noradrenergic pathways also originating in the brainstem contribute to arousal. Further, lesions to the reticular formation in the brainstem or to the three thalamic nuclei discussed above produce coma, demonstrating that these structures are necessary (but not sufficient) for arousal. In addition, drugs used in anesthesia and to aid sleep also affect RAS activity.

An additional brain structure that is important for sleep regulation is the hypothalamus. We know that the hypothalamus produces a neuropeptide, orexin (also called hypocretin), which also helps regulate sleep–wake cycles. Absence of orexin is one cause of **narcolepsy**, in which an affected person abruptly falls asleep while engaged in purposeful activity. Additionally, there are different sleep-regulating portions of the hypothalamus, with opposite effects on sleep. Some when lesioned can induce sleep, whereas others when lesioned restrict sleep.

Within a wakeful state, there are variations in level of attention, with an optimal state labeled as **vigilance** or **sustained attention**, which is supported by right-lateralized cortical (inferior parietal and frontal) and subcortical (thalamic and brainstem) regions. Noradrenergic and cholinergic projections from the brainstem to these other structures regulate sustained attention, and pharmacological manipulations of these neurotransmitters can alter performance on tasks that measure sustained attention, such as continuous performance tasks (CPTs). In a typical CPT, stimuli (e.g., numbers) flash one at a time on a screen, and the test taker must respond to a target stimulus (e.g., the number 1) or a target sequence of stimuli (e.g., 9 immediately followed by a 1) and withhold responses to other stimuli. Poor performance on CPT tasks is a hallmark of ADHD and schizophrenia (which are discussed in Chapter 10) but is also found in many other disorders, consistent with what was said earlier about the ubiquity of attention problems in various disorders that affect behavior (essentially the disorders described in this book).

The third and most cognitively important type of attention is **selective attention**, which is defined as directing attention to some things and ignoring others in order to accomplish a task. Without selective attention, virtually all goal-directed behavior would be impossible, whether it be carrying on a coherent conversation, recalling an episode, planning a trip, fixing something, finding one's way in a new place, or writing a chapter or story. Attention selection can be bottom-up, in which an object (e.g., a snake in your path) grabs attention, or top-down, in which internal goals of the human or other animal determine what aspects of the environment warrant attention. As is true for many other behavioral functions described in this book, a distributed system of subcortical and cortical brain structures implement selective attention.

Posner, Walker, Friedrich, and Rafal (1984) developed and tested an influential box-and-arrow model of this distributed system involved in selective attention. This model involves seven operations (alert, interrupt, localize, disengage, move, engage, and inhibit) involved in shifts of attention, with each operation mediated by different brain structures in the attentional network discussed earlier. They demonstrated with their spatial cueing paradigm that patients with right parietal lesions and the syndrome of attentional neglect had particular difficulty with disengaging attention, as discussed later. In contrast, patients with supranuclear palsy, which involves degeneration of the superior colliculus, as well as parts of the basal ganglia (BG), had particular trouble with moving attention. In their model, these two behaviors are interpreted as localized deficits in a particular operation. However, their approach has been challenged by connectionist models of attention, whose functional components are less localized. The Posner spatial cueing paradigm has also been used in research on other disorders of attention, such as ADHD.

TYPICAL DEVELOPMENT

Johnson and de Haan (2011) have reviewed the development of visual attention in infants. Not surprisingly, they find that not all the types of attention discussed above are present at birth. Typical newborns clearly have sleep–wake cycles and so exhibit arousal and alertness, so we can infer they are probably conscious at a basic level. They orient to unexpected stimuli (e.g., a ringing bell) and may become distressed by them, reflecting their immature capacity for state or emotion regulation. But their attention is hardly voluntary or sustained. In the Johnson and de Haan (2011) account, newborn visual attention is mostly mediated by the superior colliculus in the brainstem, with some input from deep layers 5 and 6 of primary visual cortex (V1). Newborns are capable of saccadic (not smooth, but "jagged") tracking of a moving object and preferentially orient to objects in the temporal (i.e., outer or peripheral) visual field in each eye. An important attentional phenomenon, **inhibition of return** (decreased probability of making a visual saccade to a previous target), emerges early in infancy and is thought to be mediated by the superior colliculus. Inhibition of return helps ensure that infants' scanning of the external world is complete and flexible. In the Johnson and de Haan (2011) model, by 1 month of age, infants have added inputs from layer 4 of Brodmann's area 17 and the BG to their visual attention network and these additions result in new behaviors, including **obligatory attention** and reduced peripheral orienting. Obligatory attention is an inability to disengage visual attention from a stimulus, sometimes leading to considerable distress in the infant, and can be thought of as the opposite of inhibition of return. Johnson and de Haan (2011) explain obligatory attention as being due to emerging cortical inhibition of the superior colliculus, which in effect overshoots the mark.

Voluntary attention requires cortical control and therefore inhibition of subcortical circuits, but this inhibition needs to be balanced by activation of cortically guided visual saccades. In Posner's model, discussed earlier, obligatory attention could be explained by a failure of the disengage function. As we will see, a deficit in the disengage function underlies hemispatial neglect, so obligatory attention could be viewed as a normal analogue of neglect. Obligatory attention is also interesting clinically because attentional fixedness is found in many psychiatric disorders, such as obsessive–compulsive disorder (OCD), although the neural explanation may differ. Bryson (1970) demonstrated the presence of obligatory attention in preschool children with autism several years past the age when this phenomenon ends in typically developing children.

By 2 months of age, according to the Johnson and de Haan (2011) model, more of layer 4 of Brodmann's area 17 and the ventral visual pathway in the neocortex become functional, enabling processing in the central visual and nasal (i.e., inner) fields and smooth pursuit of a moving object. Finally, by 3 to 6 months, the surface layers 2 and 3 of Brodmann's area 17 develop, as do the frontal eye fields necessary for voluntary eye movements. These neural changes enable a form of top-down selective attention, namely, anticipatory eye movements (Haith, Hazan, & Goodman, 1988). In the visual anticipation paradigm utilized by Haith et al. (1988), infants around 3 months of age quickly learn a regular right-versus-left pattern in visual presentations and are able to move their eyes to where a display will appear. In sum, in the first 6 months of life there is a gradual shift of control of visual attention from subcortical to neocortical structures with a resulting increase in voluntary control of visual attention. Improved attention partly explains substantial changes in the efficiency of visual processing over the first several months of life. The time necessary to habituate to a novel stimulus declines from 3 or 4 minutes in newborns to just a few seconds by 5 months of age. The duration of sustained attention increases and is increasingly coordinated with intentional behaviors, involving eye–hand coordination or locomotion (Berk, 2005).

Of course, as anyone who has interacted with toddlers or early-elementary-age children knows well, the development of attention is protracted well beyond infancy. Attention development postinfancy interacts with the development of language, planning, and knowledge. Sustained and selective attention reaches an optimal point for novel problem-solving tasks in late adolescence and then declines slowly after that, although knowledge and strategies can offset the losses in attentional abilities that come with normal aging.

From this brief summary of the development of attention, one can extract several constraints that can be placed on explanations of disorders of attention: (1) attention is not innate and develops in interaction with other aspects of development; (2) the development of attention is both **experience-expectant** (requires environmental inputs that are species-typical and ubiquitous, such as visual and other sensory experience but also social and language input) and **experience-dependent** (requires experiences that can vary across individuals, such as opportunities for play and problem solving and eventually formal instruction); (3) there is no single attention center in the brain, but rather a network of subcortical and cortical structures that develop at different times; and (4) attention malfunctions in typical development in ways that overlap with pathologies of attention in atypical development (e.g., obligatory attention).

DISORDERS

The two classic neurological disorders of attention that will be discussed here are **hemineglect** and **Bálint syndrome** (see reviews in Banich & Compton, 2011; Gazzaniga et al., 2009; Rafal, 1997). Both are caused by acquired lesions and do not have a known complete neurodevelopmental or psychiatric analogue, although acquired lesions in children can produce neglect (e.g., Ferro, Martins, & Tavera, 1984; Thompson, Ewing-Cobbs, Fletcher, Miner, & Levin, 1991; Trauner, Wulfeck, Tallal, & Hesselink, 2000). Hemineglect is defined as "a failure to report, respond, or orient to stimuli that are presented contralateral to a brain lesion, when this failure is not due to elementary sensory or motor disorders" (Heilman, Maher, Greenwald, & Rothi, 1997). Hemineglect is an amazing disorder to think about, because it dramatically illustrates that our conscious experience of the world can be selectively lost. For a patient with hemineglect, half the world has essentially disappeared! Bálint syndrome is a rarer and even more surprising disorder, in which consciousness of the external world is now limited to a single object. This limitation is called *simultagnosia*, the inability to attend to more than one object at a time regardless of their locations in the visual fields. As a consequence, individuals with Bálint syndrome also have impaired control of gaze direction and impaired visually guided reaching. In both hemineglect and Bálint syndrome, attention is overselective because of unbalanced competition, between attentional hemifields in neglect and between objects in Bálint syndrome. Bálint syndrome is somewhat reminiscent of obligatory attention in typical infants, in which attention becomes fixated on a single object and cannot be disengaged.

A unilateral lesion is sufficient to cause hemineglect but the occurrence of Bálint syndrome requires a bilateral lesion, usually in both parietal–occipital junctions. A consensus lesion site for hemineglect, averaged over many cases (Rafal, 1997), is the right inferior parietal lobule (Brodmann's areas 39 and 40), but the heterogeneity of neglect has led to controversy about its localization. A more recent meta-analysis found consensus for the right superior temporal gyrus, insula, and basal ganglia (Karnath, Fruhmann Berger, Kuker, & Rorden, 2004). Hillis et al. (2005) used a different method to investigate the neural substrates of neglect in a series of 50 patients with subcortical strokes that disconnected white matter underlying different cortical regions leading to hypoperfusion (reduced blood flow) in those regions. White matter lesions were measured with DTI and hypoperfusion with fMRI. They found that hypoperfusion was necessary for the behavioral symptom of neglect, and the critical cortical region varied according to whether the neglect was object based (right superior temporal gyrus) or neglect of extrapersonal space (inferior parietal lobule and temporoparietal junction), with the latter being consistent with the results reported in Rafal (1997). These somewhat different results remind us of the perils of the localization approach. Because these right temporal and parietal loci are part of a distributed network that guides spatially guided behavior, lesions elsewhere in that network can produce neglect (i.e., in dorsolateral PFC, cingulate gyrus, thalamus, and white matter connections between these structures, as the Hillis et al., 2005, study demonstrates).

There are behavioral subtypes of hemineglect, the two main ones being **attentional** and **intentional** neglect, with many patients having a combination of the two. The former is defined as a hemispatial deficit in awareness of one or all sensory modalities and the latter as an exploratory deficit in contralesional space. As might be expected, the causative lesions in the two subtypes differ, with attentional neglect being more associated with the parietal portion of the distributed network described above and intentional neglect being associated with the frontal portions of this network. As we will see below, attentional neglect is further subdivided by the spatial reference frame that is affected. Since many clinical tests of neglect involve both awareness and exploration, distinguishing these two subtypes requires tests that differentiate awareness from exploratory deficits. Several researchers have developed ingenious tasks that make this distinction, including a bisection task with a pulley device allowing the patient to move the pencil to the left with a rightward movement (Bisiach, Geminiani, Berti, & Rusconi, 1990), and a cancellation task (i.e., a task that requires the subject to cross out every target in a page of targets with distractors) in which an opaque sheet with a target-sized opening is placed over the page of targets and foils (Rafal, 1997). In the pulley task, the pencil to bisect the line could either be moved to the left with the usual leftward movement or with a rightward movement. This device should improve the performance of patients only if they have problems making movements to the left and not problems attending to the left side of space (i.e., intentional neglect), because they can move the pencil to the left to bisect the complete line they are aware of. Patients who improved line bisection performance with this rightward movement were classified as having intentional neglect. In contrast, patients who did not improve using rightward movement were considered to have attentional neglect because both movement directions still required attending to contralesional space to be aware of the entire line to be bisected. In the modified cancellation task with an opaque sheet, there are again two conditions, one in which the top sheet is moved to the left to find targets and one in which the bottom sheet is moved to the right. Again, patients with intentional neglect should improve in the second condition, whereas patients with attentional neglect should not.

There is a very rich experimental psychology of neglect in which careful experiments have helped to define the underlying operative cognitive processes. Although much more needs to be learned, these studies have demonstrated that the deficit is not absolute (due to permanent damage to one attentional or intentional field) because various manipulations can reduce or even temporarily eliminate the neglect. Also, these studies have demonstrated that patients vary in terms of which spatial reference frame is affected—an object-centered spatial reference frame versus an egocentric external spatial reference frame utilized in visual search and exploration. In object-centered neglect (see Figure 7.1), neglect occurs on the *left*

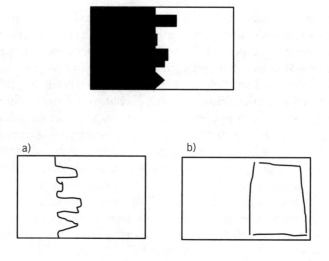

FIGURE 7.1. Object-centered neglect.

side of an object regardless of where the object is in external visual space, but not on the *right* side of an object in the usually impaired left hemifield (Driver, Baylis, & Rafal, 1993; Marshall & Halligan, 1994).

Studies of neglect patients using the Posner spatial cueing paradigm discussed earlier (Posner et al., 1984) suggest that neglect is due to a problem disengaging attention from targets in the good field rather than sensory competition among possible targets (because there are not competing targets in the Posner paradigm). Of course, there is competition at the level of disengagement itself, which is balanced in typical individuals but exhibits horizontal imbalance in neglect patients. Other research with visual search tasks has shown that this disengagement deficit is proportional to the number of distractors in the ipsilesional field (Eglin, Robertson, & Knight, 1989) and that cancellation performance improves dramatically if the patient's task is to erase all the targets (Mark, Kooistra, & Heilman, 1988). In the erasure version of the cancellation task, patients with left hemineglect initially erase targets in the intact right ipsilesional field, but once there are no more targets in that field to disengage from, they can move attention to targets in the impaired left contralesional field.

These and other studies make the important point that neglect appears to be due to unbalanced competition between the two hemispheres and that the dynamic of this competition can be shifted by manipulating task conditions. (There are other theories of neglect, including the **anisometry hypothesis** [Bisiach, Neppi-Modona, & Ricci, 2002], which holds that the representation of space itself is distorted in neglect such that the periphery of this representation is compressed.) This competition model of neglect is an example of the horizontal imbalance model discussed in Chapter 5 and later applied to some psychiatric disorders. This interpretation of neglect is consistent with the **biased-competition model** of attention (Desimone & Duncan, 1995), which holds that attention acts by biasing ongoing brain activity, either in a top-down or bottom-up fashion. This model of attention has been implemented in neural networks (O'Reilly et al., 2011).

Consistent with the competition model, neglect can be temporarily alleviated by treatments that help balance the competition between the hemispheres by increasing input to the impaired (usually right) hemisphere or by reducing input to the intact (usually left) hemisphere. These treatments include transcranial magnetic stimulation (TMS) used to disrupt activity in the good hemisphere, unilateral eye patching of the ipsilesional eye, unilateral caloric stimulation (i.e., irrigation with cold water) of the contralesional ear, and vibration of the contralesional neck muscles (Banich & Compton, 2011).

The dynamic nature of neglect makes it clear just how different it is from a simple sensory (e.g., a visual field cut or hemianopia) or motor (hemiparesis) deficit, which is more absolute but actually less impairing. Patients with a hemianopia cannot see one side of space because they are blind in that field, but they are less impaired than a neglect patient because they can scan that side of external space by moving their eyes. They do not lack awareness of a whole side of space. Similarly, patients with a hemiplegia still recognize that exploration and action are needed in the contralesional side of external space and can accomplish that with their intact limb. Neglect is a disorder of consciousness, and demonstrates dramatically that attention is spatially organized and that consciousness can have a dramatic gap in it. So the real-world clinical effects are profound. Obviously, a neglect patient should not drive or operate dangerous equipment.

CHAPTER SUMMARY

The cognitive neuroscience of attention has made important discoveries about brain regions involved in conscious experience. Disorders of attention, such as hemineglect, demonstrate that attention is spatially organized and depends on the dorsal visual stream. In neglect, there can be a partial gap in consciousness of the external world.

EXERCISES

1. Search for "hemineglect" on YouTube to watch a video of a patient with a visual neglect.

2. Using open-source software at *Neurosynth.org* enter the term "attention." The resulting image represents a meta-analysis of brain imaging studies including the term "attention": The highlighted areas represent both negative and positive correlations. Based on what was discussed in this chapter, why would the highlighted areas be implicated?

3. Now, in the "search again" box, type another normal function, such as "working memory." Use the scroll bars on the right sides of the three slice perspectives to find active brain areas associated with this function. What areas, if any, overlap with the areas implicated in attention?

CHAPTER 8

■■■■■■■

Disorders of Language

To locate the damage that destroys speech and to locate speech are two different things.
—FINGER (1994, p. 379; summary of John Hughlings Jackson, 1874)

Human language is the happy result of bringing together two systems that all higher organisms must have: A representational system and a communication system.
—MILLER (1990, p. 12)

Language is a new machine made out of old parts.
—BATES AND MCWHINNEY (1988, p. 147)

DEFINITION

The quotes above highlight some of the important issues that have been debated, sometimes intensely, in research on human language: (1) How is language mediated by the brain?, (2) How did it evolve?, (3) How is it related to other cognitive processes? We will address these issues as we present what is known about the neuroscience of typical and disordered language.

First, what is human language? It is a unique, evolved audio-vocal communication system that builds on specialized human social cognition (joint attention and intersubjectivity), that is flexible and generative enough to make virtually any conscious cognitive representation in the mind of a speaker accessible to the mind of a listener, and that requires a degree of fine motor control, a level of working memory, and possibly other cognitive processes that are found only in humans. As far as we know, human language is unique among animal communication systems because it uses symbols, exhibits compositionality, and is recursive.

"Compositionality" means that parts of a human utterance can be manipulated independently from other parts by a human language user, and "recursive" means that embedding of one clause within another (e.g., "This is the dog that chased the cat that lived in the house that faced the street that ran to the river . . . ") can generate a potentially infinite number of possible human utterances. As we will see, there are competing theories (i.e., symbolic vs. subsymbolic theories, discussed in Chapter 4) of the neural computations that underlie these properties of human language.

The definition of human language given above makes clear what some of the old parts are that went into constructing the new machine of human language and includes the insight in the quote from Miller (1963) above. Miller's (1963) insight was that human language allows the most extensive convergence of representation and communication seen in any species (although nonhuman primates, cetaceans, birds, and even prairie dogs have impressive communication systems, the range of what can be communicated is much more limited). It also makes it clear that human language must be served by a distributed system in the brain that overlaps and interacts with virtually all of cognition: perception, attention, memory, social cognition, executive control, and emotion/motivation. So, language cannot be discretely localized in the brain, although some components of language may be more localized than others. It is obvious that at least some aspects of language must be learned from experience (feral children who are not exposed to language do not learn to speak), and we will see in the section on typical development that the brain substrates of language change as it is learned, consistent with the interactive specialization theory and contrary to the notion of an innate language module. Whether there is a language module has been and continues to be a very controversial issue in the psychology of language, with Chomskyians providing theoretical arguments and evidence for such a module and connectionists countering with demonstrations of how language can be learned using generic cognitive architectures.

How did language evolve? Of course, we do not know and will probably never know. But we can lay out some requirements for the evolution of human language. First, it is built on the evolved human social cognition needed for successful functioning in large, extended kinship groups that engage in many cooperative activities (e.g., hunting, foraging, child-rearing, fighting, and trading with other kinship groups). Second, it thus co-evolved with cultural evolution.

A more direct form of co-evolution was important in many other human adaptations (e.g., domestication of plants and animals co-evolved with lactose, gluten, and canine tolerance in some, but not all, early human groups). In these examples of co-evolution, both humans and the relevant plant or animal evolved (i.e., incorporated useful mutations into their genomes) as domestication proceeded. Of course, by "canine tolerance," I do not mean eating dogs, but rather incorporating dogs into human social groups, first as guards and then as pets. It has been demonstrated that dogs, even young puppies, have adaptations in social cognition that foster their interaction with (exploitation of) humans that are not found in wolves or chimps (Tomasello & Kaminski, 2009). It is an interesting question whether humans have correspondingly evolved adaptations that foster interactions with dogs, and if so, whether such human adaptations could now be innate.

The distinct kind of co-evolution of human language and culture arose because language itself facilitated a new kind of evolution, cultural evolution, which proceeds much faster than biological evolution, and whose acceleration, both for good and for bad, we are still experiencing today. Early prelanguage humans were likely already participating in cultural evolution using other means of social transmission (i.e., imitation), but the emergence of language greatly facilitated the transmission of culture. The co-evolution of human culture and language required evolutionary modifications of several "old parts": the vocal tract and articulatory control, social cognition, working memory, and very likely many others. Most importantly, the length of the developmental period had to evolve to permit language and cultural acquisition by human children, who have the longest period of development of any species. These and other ideas about the evolution of language have been discussed at length by various scholars (e.g., Donald, 2001; Lieberman, 2002; see Pinker, 1995, for a somewhat different view).

Turning from this evolutionary perspective, linguists define language in terms of its components (see Table 8.1). The structure of language is hierarchical: smaller units (phonemes) are combined into units of meaning (morphemes) contained in a **lexicon**, which are combined in a lawful way (through **syntax**), into phrases and sentences, which have meaning (**semantics**). The five components of phonemes, morphemes, lexicon, syntax, and semantics comprise what is called basic "structural" language.

Structural language is distinguished from the last two components in the table, **prosody** and **discourse**, which are concerned with the social use of language. But as soon as we require that the meanings of structural language be intersubjective, which they are in all typical language use, the distinction between structural language and its social use gets blurred. In other words, because the phrases and sentences of a language allow the speaker to refer to a present, past, or imagined state of affairs that can be

TABLE 8.1. Components of a Sound-Based Language

Phonemes	Individual sounds in words that make a difference in their meaning (e.g., /b/ vs. /d/ in pairs of words like "bog" vs. "dog.").
Morphemes	Combinations of phonemes that make a meaningful word or part of a word (in sign languages, the equivalent of a morpheme is a visuomotor sign).
Syntax	Possible ways of combining morphemes into words, phrases, and sentences (called "grammar," in popular usage) in a particular language.
Lexicon	The set of all words in a given language known by an individual language user in a kind of "mental dictionary" including their pronunciations, spelling (only in a written language), and grammatical forms, but *not* their meanings, unlike a real dictionary.
Semantics	The meanings assigned to morphemes, phrases, and sentences.
Prosody	The vocal intonation and stress pattern that can modify the literal meaning of words and sentences.
Discourse	The linking of sentences such that they constitute a narrative or conversation.

shared with a listener, successful communication always requires that the speaker monitor whether the listener knows what the speaker is referring to, which is called "securing reference." How infants learn about securing reference is an important question in the development of language.

These linguistic definitions have often been taken to imply that each component of structural language is actually cognitively separate from the others when language is processed in a real human brain, and some theories of language processing make that claim. But recent evidence indicates these components interact extensively and bidirectionally in language processing (e.g., the model of the word superiority effect discussed in Chapter 4). We can readily grasp the importance of interactive and bidirectional processing if we compare our ability to perceive familiar versus unfamiliar spoken words in sentences in a noisy background. Our top-down lexical semantic and syntactic expectations help to rescue a familiar word from noise, but not an unfamiliar one. Because of this bidirectional interactivity, we should not expect clean dissociations in either typical language processing or in disorders, either developmental or acquired. For instance, research has shown developmental links between grammar and the lexicon (Bates & Goodman, 1997) and between grammatical morphology and speech perception (Joanisse, 2007). As explained later, close links have also been demonstrated between phonological and lexical development. So the emerging picture is that there are dependencies among the four components of structural language in Table 8.1 in both typical and atypical development. We also know that speech perception and production (phonological development) leads development of the other three components. As we will see later, phonological deficits are a core feature of developmental disorders of speech and language, so explaining what causes these deficits is a key scientific goal of research on these disorders. Finally, as the last two components in Table 8.1 make clear, language is broader than basic structural language, and I turn next to these two other levels of language processing.

Combinations of sentences into a narrative or exposition constitute a **discourse**. Discourse processing encompasses both the production and the comprehension of discourses, and requires additional general cognitive processes not required by the comprehension of single sentences or phrases. These additional cognitive processes include making inferences and linking the elements of the discourse into a coherent mental representation. Discourse processing places additional demands on attention and working memory beyond what is required for processing single sentences, and also depend more heavily on the listener's store of prior knowledge relevant to the topic of the discourse (see Kintsch, 1994). Discourse processing makes it very clear that language and other aspects of cognition cannot be totally separate from each other. In our real everyday use of language, we are nearly always processing discourses. Because of the additional cognitive demands of discourse processing, its development takes much longer than the development of basic structural language and depends in modern societies on formal education. Much of formal education is devoted to learning a *written* language and learning to produce and comprehend it, a task which continues through college, graduate school, and beyond in "knowledge" workers. Thus, we should expect to find disorders of discourse processing in the absence of deficits in basic structural language. As is discussed later in this chapter, that is indeed the case.

Finally, we come to **prosody**, which is considered a paralinguistic or pragmatic aspect of language, meaning that it is added to structural language and discourse. Prosody is the intonation with which a word or sentence is uttered. Think of at least three different prosodies, and hence meanings, you can impart to this sentence: "What is this thing called love?" (*Hint*: It is fine to change the punctuation, even substituting an "!"

for "?.") Other aspects of pragmatic language are gestures, postures, and facial expressions. We know from our own everyday experiences and from professional mimes that these nonverbal, pragmatic features of language are richly communicative by themselves. Given appropriate social cognition (intersubjectivity) and pragmatics, a lot can be communicated without words, perhaps giving us a glimpse of what human communication was like before the evolution of structural language. There are acquired disorders of prosody (e.g., the aprosodias). Some developmental disorders include altered prosody in their presentation (e.g., autism).

BRAIN MECHANISMS

Given the interactivity among the components of language defined in Table 8.1, we should expect that these processes are not as discretely localized as the classical aphasia model predicted (see Figure 8.3 and Table 8.3 on p. 118). A large meta-analysis of more than 100 imaging studies of phonology, semantics, and sentence or text processing (Vigneau et al., 2006) found that peak activity for these three components largely overlapped in the left hemisphere, with peaks for each found in *both* anterior and posterior sites, and in *both* classic perisylvian language areas and in surrounding areas in parietal, temporal, and frontal cortex. So, it appears that components of language processing are distributed rather than localized in human adults.

There are also more direct demonstrations of such interactions in neuroimaging studies of language. For instance, Friederici, von Cramon, and Kotz (2007) demonstrated an interaction between left-hemisphere syntactic processing and right-hemisphere prosodic processing in the comprehension of ambiguous sentences such as the one discussed earlier ("What is this thing called love?"). This interaction is mediated by white matter connections between the two hemispheres.

TYPICAL DEVELOPMENT

Clearly children do not speak at birth (the word "infant" literally means "without speech"), so speech and language must develop somehow. How they develop has been a focus of intense investigation and debate in the field of psychology for many decades. The paradigm of behaviorism that dominated academic psychology for most of the first half of the 20th century held that language was acquired like all behavior, that is, by learning stimulus–response (S-R) associations. This empiricist approach to language acquisition was severely challenged by Noam Chomsky's (1959) long review of B. F. Skinner's book *Verbal Behavior* (Skinner, 1957). Chomsky identified several aspects of human language that he argued were unlearnable not only by means of S-R associations, but by any purely inductive process. So, Chomsky was a realist or idealist in the sense defined earlier, and like other realists in the history of philosophy, he argued that there must be innate ideas that cannot be learned from experience.

There are several key parts of Chomsky's unlearnability argument. First, he argued that the language children are exposed to is not rich enough to support the language structures they actually acquire (called the "poverty of the stimulus" argument). Second, he argued that S-R associations would not support a key property of human language, namely the already-discussed property of recursion (the ability to embed phrases within phrases to generate new utterances). Recursion requires dependencies among nonadjacent words in a phrase or sentence, and it was not clear how an S-R association could capture such dependencies. Third, he argued that human language was unlearnable with any extant computational mechanism. This argument holds that learning grammatical rules is analogous to trying to learn a concept from only positive instances, not from a mix of positive and negative instances with clear feedback about which instances are incorrect. Infants generally hear only grammatical speech; they are not exposed to instances of ungrammatical speech that are clearly marked as such. Without such negative feedback, it is much harder to constrain the space of possible hypotheses (see discussion in Bishop, 1997). Since language was evidently unlearnable, Chomsky argued that there must be innate and universal language structures (an innate language acquisition device [LAD]) that guide an infant's language learning. Regardless of which human language an infant was exposed to, the LAD would permit its acquisition. So, Chomsky's theory posits an innate, modular, and maturational view of language acquisition, a view that would seem to require an innate LAD in the brain.

Chomsky was very influential in launching the cognitive revolution in psychology, which was dominated by the symbolic paradigm discussed in Chapter 4. As discussed in that chapter, the symbolic paradigm takes its view of mental computations from formal or symbolic logic developed in the field of mathematics. The human mind is viewed as a symbol-processing machine that operates by rules that define how one proposition can be transformed into another. The referential content (semantics) of the propositions does not matter, and that content could be replaced by algebraic variables (e.g., x, y, and z). What counts are the relations among variables. So, in this view of cognition generally, and language specifically, what really matters is syntax and the logical operations that act on syntactic structures to produce new propositions or sentences. The other components of language, such as phonology and lexical semantics, are viewed as less important.

Chomsky's view dominated the field of language development for several decades and also stimulated a whole new field of research into children's language development (e.g., Brown, 1973). As is often the case in scientific research, eventually stubborn facts about children's language development emerged that challenged Chomsky's highly influential theory (or, one could even say, *paradigm*). Two key discoveries were (1) that connectionist networks *could* learn linguistic regularities and exhibit rule-like linguistic behavior, without having the explicit linguistic rules postulated by Chomsky's theory, and (2) that actual human infants were capable of statistical learning of linguistic regularities (E. M. Saffran, Aslin, & Newport, 1996; J. R. Saffran, 2003). These discoveries directly contradicted Chomsky's (un)learnability argument: the stimulus was rich enough to support learning, and the learning mechanism was powerful enough to accomplish that learning. Much of this work with connectionist models and statistical learning focused on the acquisition of syntax, partly because syntax was so central to Chomsky's theory. Models were developed that acquired the English past tense (Elman et al., 1997; Marchman, Plunkett, & Goodman, 1997), speech, and reading.

Figures 8.1 and 8.2 depict two such models, the first of the development of speech and language, and the second, the development of single-word reading, with reading building on oral language skills developed earlier. As discussed in Pennington and Bishop (2009), in developing an oral language, one of the first tasks an infant must master is the perception and production of the speech sounds specific to the native language (Kuhl, 2004). Although innate constraints influence some aspects of human language acquisition (e.g., Pinker, 1999), mastering a particular oral, and especially written, language requires extensive learning, much of it implicit statistical learning (Saffran et al., 1996). In statistical learning, which is similar to what is called procedural learning (discussed in Chapter 9) and probabilistic learning (discussed in Chapter 10), the subject unconsciously learns the statistical dependencies between adjacent items in a string of stimuli. These dependencies could define an artificial grammar or word boundaries in a continuous string of phonemes, both of which a human infant acquiring a particular language must learn. Consequently, connectionist models, which implement statistical learning of speech, language, and reading, provide a useful framework for thinking about

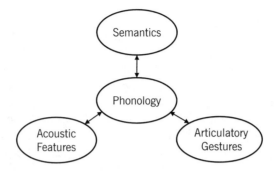

FIGURE 8.1. Connectionist model of speech and language. Based on Guenther (1995), Joanisse (2000), and Westermann and Miranda (2004).

relations among language impairment (LI), reading disability (RD), and speech-sound disorder (SSD) at the cognitive level (see Figures 8.1 and 8.2). Both of these figures display in simple fashion "triangle" models in which circles are layers of many artificial neurons and arrows are the multiple, bidirectional connections between layers of neurons (see Chapter 4). So, even though Figures 8.1 and 8.2 superficially resemble box-and-arrow models, the actual connectionist models have many more nodes and connections and are actually implemented on a computer.

The development of speech production (Figure 8.1) has been depicted in several computational models (Guenther, 1995; Joanisse, 2000; Joanisse, 2004; Joanisse, 2007; Joanisse & Seidenberg, 2003; Markey, 1994; Menn, Markey, Mozer, & Lewis, 1993; Plaut & Kello, 1999; Westermann & Miranda, 2004). The difficult developmental task

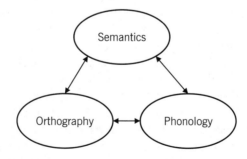

FIGURE 8.2. Connectionist model of reading acquisition (e.g., Harm & Seidenberg, 1999).

these models address is how young children learn the complex mapping between acoustic features and articulatory gestures, particularly when important aspects of the articulatory gestures made by adult models are not observable. For example, it is difficult for children to observe the placement of an adult's tongue while producing the "th" sound. Babbling almost certainly supplements imitation in learning these mappings. In these computational models, intermediate units learn the particular abstract mappings between acoustic features and articulatory gestures, and the representations of these abstract mappings are phonological representations. However, these models do not explain clinical cases where phonological representations develop without speech (e.g., anarthric children with oral reading skills; Bishop, 1985).

We will next cover phonological development in more detail because it is so crucial for understanding developmental disorders of speech and language, including SSD, LI, and RD. As discussed earlier, phonology concerns the sounds of a spoken language, which vary across human languages. Before children learn the words in a language (lexical morphemes) or how to combine them (syntax), they begin learning the sounds specific to the language they hear. This learning actually begins in the womb in the third trimester. Infants can hear speech in the womb, particularly its melody or prosody, so they prefer the sound of their mother's voice at birth. This prenatal learning also affects their early vocal productions. The prosody of crying in neonates differs as a function of the language they heard in utero. Mampe, Friederici, Christophe, and Wermke (2009) found that the prosody of neonatal crying was different in French versus German babies, with the neonates in each group matching their crying to the prosody of the language they heard in the womb.

In the Chomskyan paradigm, knowledge of phonemes was considered innate, and so a newborn possessed, in some sense, *all* the phonemes in *all* the world's languages (otherwise Chomsky's theory would have no way of accounting for successful language acquisition by international adoptees). Hence, learning the phonology of the infant's native language was simply a process of selecting the subset of phonemes specific to that language. In this paradigm, babbling by infants was not considered to be important to the infant's phonological development (see review in Mareschal et al., 2007). In Jakobson's (1941) classical work on phonological development, phonology was viewed as independent from babbling, in part because there appeared to be a discontinuity between the end of babbling and the appearance of speech. A second argument for the independence of babbling and phonology is found in Lenneberg's (1967) influential book on language development. Lenneberg reasoned that since babbling is similar in both deaf and hearing infants, it could not be important for their spoken word productions, which differ markedly.

As discussed in Mareschal et al. (2007), more careful observations disproved both the discontinuity between babbling and speech and the supposed similarity of babbling in deaf and hearing infants. It turns out that babbling in deaf infants is actually delayed in its onset and different in its sounds once it appears. Both Jakobson's and Lenneberg's arguments for the independence of babbling from phonology can be seen as examples of how one's theoretical paradigm (i.e., phonemes are innate) influences how data are interpreted.

Empirical studies of infants' and children's phonological development have seriously questioned (1) whether phonemes are innate, (2) whether learning phonology is simply a process of selection, and (3) whether babbling is unimportant in that learning (Mareschal et al., 2007). Instead, research supports the view that infants learn to produce phonology of their native language through statistical learning. In this learning process, babbling is a self-teaching device through which the child learns the very complex mapping between acoustic features and articulatory gestures, a feat that at first blush *does* seem truly unlearnable. Children clearly imitate the speech they hear, just as they learn many other things by imitation, but in imitating speech they must copy many articulatory gestures that they cannot see (those that occur inside the mouth and vocal tract). How can they work around this seemingly insuperable barrier? They do this by imitating ambient language sounds and then practice them by imitating *themselves* in babbling. Even if they cannot watch their own articulatory gestures, each gesture has a distinct proprioceptive and motor "signature." Through repetitive babbling with slight variations, infants slowly learn the complex mapping between acoustic features and articulatory gestures appropriate for their native language. In this process, both perception and production of speech sounds changes from a universal pattern seen in infants across languages to one that is more specific to the native language.

Production in babbling changes in the first year of life, and begins with isolated vowel sounds before 6 months of age. At around 6 months, canonical babbling appears, with infants producing long strings of repeated consonant–vowel (CV) syllables (e.g., "gagagaga . . ."). Similar to perceptual development, the vowel space of babbling productions is gradually assimilated to the ambient language, a process that has been linked to the increasing capacity for vocal imitation (Kuhl & Meltzoff, 1996).

Regarding the infant's development of speech *perception*, between 6 and 12 months of age, infants gradually lose the ability to discriminate non-native phonemes (Werker & Tees, 1984). However, this loss is not simply one of de-selection of non-native contrasts, as the Chomskyan selectionist theory would suggest. If that theory were correct, infants would lose the ability to make *all* non-native contrasts. Instead, Best and colleagues have shown that there is a gradient of performance with non-native contrasts, depending on how they map onto native contrasts (Best, McRoberts, & Goodell, 2001). So, rather than selecting and deselecting from an innate, universal set of phonemes, developing infants assimilate their babbling to match the ambient language, losing some but not all non-native contrasts in the process. Kuhl (1991) has demonstrated a similar phenomenon in vowel perception, such that infants exposed to different languages develop different vowel contrasts, with different attractors or prototypes.

So, perception and production of speech sounds change in tandem in the first year of life to match the ambient native language, and babbling appears to be a crucial self-teaching device in this developmental process. The development of phonological representations through babbling has been simulated in neural networks (e.g., Westermann & Miranda, 2004), providing additional evidence that phonological representations can be learned through babbling.

Infants are developing phonological representations through statistical learning in the first year of life, but much more phonological development lies ahead of them as they map phonology onto lexical semantics to acquire a spoken vocabulary in the second year of life and beyond. In this process, there appears to be a reciprocal relation between phonological and vocabulary development. Phonology and phonological memory enable the child to perform "fast mappings" of new names onto already acquired concepts, but the expanding lexicon forces the child to make new phonological distinctions in a process called lexical restructuring of phonology (Walley, 1993). Several researchers (e.g., Nittrouer, 1996) have demonstrated the protracted nature of phonological development into toddlerhood and beyond with carefully designed speech perception tasks.

The research presented here is consistent with the view that phonological representations are constructed and change to capture an optimal mapping among acoustic features, the child's vocabulary, and articulatory gestures. So, phonological representations change with spoken language development and then change further as a child learns a written language (Morais, Cary, Alegria, & Bertelson, 1979).

Taking a step back, we can see that there is an analogy between the development of visual object perception, discussed in Chapter 6, and development of speech perception (and production). Both involve perceptual organization or the construction of perceptual categories out of lower-level perceptual features (Nittrouer & Pennington, 2010). Visual objects are processed by the ventral visual pathway and auditory "objects" (e.g., spoken words) are processed by the ventral auditory pathway (with the dorsal auditory pathway being concerned with the spatial localization of auditory stimuli). Table 8.2 elaborates this analogy between visual object perception and speech perception by listing parallel phenomena in each domain. As will be discussed later, problems in speech perception in developmental disorders like dyslexia, SSD, and LI can be thought of as a kind of developmental auditory agnosia (or dysgnosia) in which the development of phonological categories is less precise than in typical development.

As described in Chapter 6 on disorders of perception, a visual object is an abstract representation that is constructed using perceptual grouping principles (the first row in Table 8.2) out of visual "stuff," such as lines, edges, angles, shading, and color, that is processed in cortical areas V1 and V2 in the occipital lobe. Similarly, an auditory object such as a speech sound is constructed using auditory grouping principles out of lower-level auditory dimensions processed by the primary and secondary auditory areas in the temporal lobe. Several experimental phenomena in speech perception demonstrate this perceptual grouping, namely duplex

TABLE 8.2. Comparison of Visual Object Perception and Speech Perception

	Visual	Speech
Perceptual grouping	Gestalt principles, etc.	Duplex perception, phoneme migration, verbal transformation effect, McGurk effect
Perceptual constancy	Across orientations, contexts, sizes, brightness	Across speakers, rates and volume of speech, contexts
Perceptual completion	Despite occlusion or visual masking	Phonemic restoration of incomplete signal. Speech perception survives auditory masking by background noise, foreign accents, or filtering (vocoded, and sine-wave speech).
Top-down effects	Categorical perception, semantic and familiarity effects	Categorical perception, semantic and familiarity effects

perception (Rand, 1974), phoneme migration, and the verbal transformation effect. Duplex perception is elicited in a dichotic listening paradigm in which one ear is presented a nonspeech chirp, and the other ear is presented a syllable that has been artificially manipulated to remove auditory information similar to the chirp. The listener perceives a complete syllable via perceptual integration *and* a chirp (duplex perception). In other words, duplex perception means that the chirp is heard both as part of a normal speech syllable and as a separate sound. Phoneme migration refers to the transposition of phonemes in spoonerisms or in different recall tasks (lists of pseudosounds) and is taken as evidence that phonemes are units of speech perception constructed from lower-level auditory dimensions. The verbal transformation effect (Warren, 1961) refers to an auditory illusion that arises when a listener hears a clearly pronounced word or phrase repeated over and over again and then perceives illusory changes in the stimulus, such as words that rhyme with the stimulus or even extreme phonetic distortions. As in visual illusions (e.g., the Necker cube) that support two different perceptions, the verbal transformation effect illustrates the operation of grouping principles that can change the percept. Finally, the McGurk effect (McGurk & MacDonald, 1976) is another illusion that illustrates the interaction between hearing and vision in speech perception. The illusion is quite dramatic and occurs when an auditory repeated syllable *ba* is paired with a video of a speaker's lips making the movement of the syllable *ga*. Instead of perceiving either *ba* or *ga*, most typical individuals perceive an illusory *da*. This illusion demonstrates that speech perception is multimodal and involves perceptual integration across input modalities.

The McGurk effect is analogous to another illusion produced by cross-modal integration, the rubber hand illusion (Botvinick & Cohen, 1998). In the rubber hand illusion, participants sees a rubber hand in a position similar to that of their own hand, which is out of view. Both their own hand and the rubber hand are stroked simultaneously with a fine brush. After about a minute of watching the rubber hand being stroked, about two-thirds of participants experience the illusion that the rubber hand is part of their body. The illusion is explained as the cross-modal integration of sight (seeing the rubber hand being stroked) and touch (simultaneously feeling their own hand being stroked).

The next two rows in Table 8.2, perceptual constancy and perceptual completion, demonstrate that like visual perception, speech perception is abstract and robust. That is, it exhibits perceptual invariance, and the abstract speech percept acts as a kind of attractor that survives a partial or masked input.

Finally, as in the word superiority effect, both object and speech perception exhibit top-down effects in which the percept is categorical even though the input is continuous. Bartlett (1932) demonstrated this categorical perception of visual objects by incrementally "morphing" a picture of a rabbit into a duck. In Bartlett's demonstration, subjects exposed to individual items in a sequence perceived each item as either a rabbit or a duck, not as a hybrid. There are many other examples of categorical visual perception in the literature (e.g., Campbell, Pascalis, Coleman, Wallace, & Benson, 1997; Newell & Bulthoff, 2002). Similarly, Liberman, Harris, Hoffman, and Griffith (1957) demonstrated a similar phenomenon in speech perception by incrementally changing one spoken syllable (e.g., *ba*) into another (e.g., *ga*). Again, subjects perceive intermediate tokens categorically as either *ba* or *ga*, thus assimilating them to a preexisting schema or category.

In sum, speech perception is like visual object perception because both involve integration of features or dimensions of the input into an abstract percept. More research is needed on how this process goes awry in developmental disorders of speech and language, which are discussed later. We now turn to the development of language lateralization in the brain.

Although development typically results by adulthood in a left-hemisphere specialization for structural language and a right-hemisphere specialization for prosody, these specializations are not present at birth. Indeed, there is remarkable plasticity in the neural substrates for language, which is demonstrated by studies of both typical development and experiments of nature. Using a new method of collecting imaging data from sleeping infants, Redcay, Haist, and Courchesne (2008) demonstrated bilateral distributed language processing in younger children (2 years old) as contrasted with less distributed, more left lateralized processing in older (3-year-old) children. This result is consistent with an interactive specialization model of language development and inconsistent with an innate or maturational account of the left-hemisphere specialization for language. As discussed in more detail in Johnson and de Haan (2011), two natural experiments are also pertinent to the question of how the left-hemisphere specialization for language develops: (1) case studies of early unilateral acquired lesions (Bates & Roe, 2001), and (2) visual language in the congenitally deaf (Neville & Bavelier, 2002).

The basic findings from infants with early unilateral lesions are that (1) either left- *or* right-hemisphere lesions disrupt early language development but not permanently, as would occur after left-hemisphere acquired lesions in adults, and (2) early right-hemisphere lesions impair comprehension more than early left-hemisphere lesions, again in contrast to what is seen in adults. Although these infants with early unilateral lesions do not reach the level of language development (or IQ) of typical controls, their language functioning is still within normal limits (i.e., they do not have LI, which is discussed later). As Neville and colleagues have shown (Neville & Bavelier, 2002), the development of sign language in the congenitally deaf also demonstrates the remarkable plasticity of the developing brain. In this case, visual language processing of signs is mapped onto unused *auditory* cortex.

Of course, there has to be some reason that language ends up lateralized to the left hemisphere in the large majority of typical adults, but there are several possibilities besides the innate or maturational explanation. For instance, some initial perceptual or motor bias in the left hemisphere could lead to gradual lateralization of language to the left hemisphere through a competitive process similar to that documented in the development of other brain specializations (e.g., ocular dominance columns). We have other evidence of left-hemisphere specialization for precise fine-motor coordination.

ACQUIRED DISORDERS OF LANGUAGE

Acquired disorders of language are called **aphasias**, and like other higher-order disorders covered in this book, such as neglect, agnosia, and amnesia, aphasias are problems in a higher-order function (language) that are not explained by a lower-level motor or sensory disorder. So by definition, aphasia cannot be due to a hearing or motor problem. Problems in speech production caused by damaged motor pathways in the articulatory system are called **dysarthria** and those caused by impairment in preprogramming the motor sequences of speech are called **dyspraxia**, and both are conceptually distinct from aphasia.

As discussed in Chapters 3 and 5, aphasia is the oldest topic in the history of neuropsychology and behavioral neurology, and models of aphasia have been at the center of developments and debates in these fields. Although the classical model of aphasia is still presented in most texts, it is important to realize that the field has made considerable progress since the classical model was proposed, and the validity of the classical subtypes has been seriously questioned by subsequent research (e.g., Caplan, 2003; Schwartz, 1984).

One can view aphasia research as a persisting debate about the validity of subtypes and the localization method itself. The contrasting deficit profiles in Broca's versus Wernicke's aphasia constituted the first double dissociation in the history of neuropsychology, but *exactly* what two components of language processing are distinguished by this double dissociation has been unclear since the outset, and ideas about the identity of the two contrasting components have evolved since then. This confusion was inevitable, since the contrast between Broca's and Wernicke's aphasia was based on *symptoms* readily observed by a clinician (fluency vs. comprehension of speech), and not on a theory of the components of language processing. As discussed earlier in Chapter 3, symptoms do not necessarily individuate or localize functions. As the field tried to move beyond symptoms to theoretically defined language functions, the double dissociation between Broca's and Wernicke's aphasias broke down.

Even though Broca and Wernicke based their subtypes on symptoms, they hypothesized underlying deficits in component functions of language processing that explained these symptoms. They conceived of Broca's area as the brain location for the "motor images of words" and Wernicke's area as the brain location for the "auditory images of words." In modern terminology, we would say "output phonology" and "input phonology," respectively. As we will see, both the functional and anatomical definitions of Broca's and Wernicke's areas have evolved due to subsequent research and theory. This evolution was virtually inevitable given the crudity of both the behavioral and neuroanatomical research methods available in the 19th century. Modern linguistics and cognitive psychology did not exist, and the only neuroimaging method was an autopsy. Why textbooks (including this one) still dutifully present the classical model is an interesting question in the history of science. The explanation may be the appealing simplicity of the classical model and the lack of a broadly accepted new paradigm.

Table 8.3 presents the classical model of aphasia, which is based on the work of Wernicke and Lichtheim in the 19th century and was revived and refined by Geschwind in the mid-20th century. To understand this model, it is useful to begin with Wernicke's model of speech production, discussed in Chapter 5 as elaborated by Lichtheim (see Figure 8.3). Wernicke's original model proposes two language centers: one for speech output, or "the motor images of words" (Broca's area in the left inferior frontal gyrus), and one for speech input, or "the auditory images of words" (Wernicke's area in the posterior left temporal lobe overlapping with the planum temporale), as well as the white matter pathway connecting these two centers (the arcuate fasciculus). Lichtheim added a Concept Center to Wernicke's original model to account for other subtypes of aphasia. In Wernicke's original model, selective damage to each of these

TABLE 8.3. Wernicke's and Broca's Classical Model of Aphasia

	Fluency	Comprehension	Repetition
Normal	+	+	+
Broca's aphasia	–	+	–
Wernicke's aphasia	+	–	–
Conduction aphasia	+	+	–
Global aphasia	–	–	–

Note. +, intact function; –, impaired function.

three components produces three different behavioral subtypes of aphasia: **Broca's aphasia, Wernicke's aphasia,** and **conduction aphasia.**

Behavioral subtypes in Wernicke's model are defined crudely by modern standards of neuropsychological testing. The 19th-century neurologist used simple bedside tests to determine if a particular language function was intact or impaired (+ or – in Table 8.3). So, for instance, speech
perception itself was not evaluated (and the means for doing so were
developed much later). Instead, classical (and contemporary) neurologists
relied on simple measures of language comprehension, thus conflating the
constructs of speech perception and language comprehension.

In Wernicke's original model, Broca's aphasia impairs speech fluency
(speech is halting and telegraphic) because the center for speech production

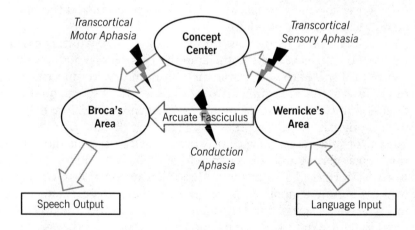

FIGURE 8.3. The Wernicke–Lichtheim model of language processing.

is damaged, but comprehension is intact because Wernicke's area is not damaged. Repetition is necessarily impaired by the problem with speech production. In contrast, Wernicke's aphasia impairs language comprehension, but spares speech fluency because Broca's area is not damaged. Absent language comprehension to monitor one's own speech, patients with Wernicke's aphasia produce fluent but empty speech, filled with naming errors (paraphasias) and jargon. Lacking comprehension (and presumably, verbal short-term memory [STM]), repetition is impaired again, but for a different reason, namely the sentence to be repeated has not been processed properly and is not held accurately in verbal STM to guide repetition. Finally, in conduction aphasia, only repetition is impaired, but fluency and comprehension are intact. The intact Wernicke's area of a patient with conduction aphasia can accurately perceive speech and comprehend speech. The patient's intact Broca's area could repeat it fluently, *if* it received the sentence from Wernicke's area. But it cannot receive it because of damage to the connection between them (the arcuate fasciculus), hence disconnection. As discussed in Chapter 5, Wernicke's description of conduction aphasia is the first example of a **disconnection** syndrome in the history of neuropsychology and neurology.

You may have noticed that the kinds of repetition errors observed in each of these three classical aphasia subtypes should be different according to this model (telegraphic in Broca's aphasia, fluent but empty in Wernicke's aphasia, and absent in Conduction aphasia), but texts describing these aphasias rarely describe the kinds of repetition errors made. Finally, a fourth, mixed subtype of aphasia is explained by Wernicke's original model, namely, **global aphasia**, in which there is damage to both Broca's and Wernicke's areas, with consequent deficits in all three aspects of language in Table 8.3.

To help deal with omission of semantics from Wernicke's model, Lichtheim added a concept or semantic center, with connections to both Wernicke's area and Broca's area (Figure 8.3). The addition of a concept center is an attempt, albeit crude, to account for language comprehension apart from speech perception. As discussed earlier, Wernicke's original model conflated speech perception and language comprehension. According to this expanded Wernicke–Lichthem model, three additional subtypes of aphasia were possible, involving either disconnection from the concept center or direct damage to it. These three subtypes are **transcortical motor aphasia**, **transcortical sensory aphasia**, and **transcortical mixed aphasia** (not depicted in Figure 8.3), with the first involving disconnection from the concept center to Broca's area, the second involving disconnection from Wernicke's area to the concept center, and the last involving damage to the concept center itself. Repetition is preserved in all three transcortical aphasias because the perisylvian language loop encompassed by Wernicke's original model is preserved. But fluency, comprehension, or both are disrupted due to disconnection from or damage to the concept center.

Obviously, a discrete, localized concept center does not make sense given what we now understand about how concepts are stored in the brain, but Lichtheim added this concept center to account for aphasic patients who did not fit Wernicke's original model, *instead* of questioning the model itself. As discussed in Chapter 3, it is a common practice in the history of science to protect an accepted paradigm by adding components to it to accommodate new data. But if there is a fundamental flaw in the paradigm, this practice is inherently degenerative and eventually leads to the collapse of the paradigm. In Chapter 3, we discussed what some of the fundamental flaws were in the localizationist program of the diagram makers, and how these eventually led to the (temporary) collapse of the paradigm in the early 20th century. We may say "temporary" because this paradigm was revived by Geschwind and others in the mid-20th century, and the aphasia subtypes in Table 8.3 are still presented in virtually every text that covers the topic of aphasia. They are even still taught to neurologists, who use these subtypes clinically to describe their patients. So, we should ask what subsequent research has taught us about the validity of Wernicke's and Lichtheim's model and the aphasia subtypes described in Table 8.3.

The original double dissociation between output and input phonology hypothesized by Broca and Wernicke evolved in the 20th century into a double dissociation between syntax (impaired in Broca's aphasia) and the lexicon (impaired in Wernicke's aphasia). This evolution seems to have been driven more by linguistic theory than by empirical observation, since Chomsky's theory emphasized the importance of syntax and its independence from lexical semantics. But then later research found flaws in this double dissociation and in the presumed independence of syntax and the lexicon (Bates & Goodman, 1997).

Kolb and Whishaw (1990) reviewed evidence bearing on the validity of the Wernicke–Lichtheim model of language and aphasia, including evidence from brain stimulation studies of the exposed left hemisphere prior to neurosurgery and analyses of a series of cases with left-hemisphere lesions. Their conclusions were that (1) stimulation of anterior or posterior language regions produces remarkably similar disruptions of language functions (consistent with the Vigneau et al., 2006, neuroimaging meta-analysis discussed earlier); (2) these stimulation effects extend well beyond the classical Broca's and Wernicke's areas; (3) there are marked individual differences in the effects of stimulation at a given point, which is consistent with the developmental plasticity for language substrates discussed earlier; (4) there is a striking convergence between the stimulation and lesion results, anterior and posterior, with both identifying similar distributed regions; (5) in the lesion cases, there was little evidence of a distinctive anterior versus posterior aphasia; (6) aphasia can also be produced by lesions of the left insular cortex and by subcortical lesions in either the thalamus or basal ganglia (BG); and (7) isolated damage to Broca's area does not produce a lasting aphasia.

In fact, Broca's original patients (whose brains were preserved) also had subcortical damage in the BG underlying Broca's area. These converging results from stimulation and lesion studies clearly do not support the Wernicke–Lichtheim model of language and aphasia (Figure 8.3), because component language functions are less localized than that model indicated and include brain regions, both cortical and subcortical, that were not included in that model.

Other researchers have noted problems with this classical aphasia model. Brown (1972) found no convincing evidence of complete independence of expressive and receptive language syndromes, and later psycholinguistic studies of patients with Broca's aphasia found they had receptive agrammatism, that is, clear deficits in comprehending syntax (Shallice, 1988). Consistent with research on acquired and developmental dyslexia, Marshall (1986) pointed out that many cases of aphasia presented with mixed symptom profiles and that only 60% fit into established syndromes. Caplan (2003) provides a good review of the problems with the classical aphasia model and the current state of aphasia research.

DEVELOPMENTAL DISORDERS OF SPEECH AND LANGUAGE

The following review is based on Pennington and Bishop (2009). The essential defining characteristics of the three disorders discussed here—language impairment (LI), reading disability (RD), and speech-sound disorder (SSD)—are summarized in Table 8.4. In each case, the disorder involves an unexpected difficulty in one aspect of development that cannot readily be explained by such factors as low intelligence or sensory–motor impairment. All three disorders lack a sharp dividing line between impairment and normality; thus, diagnosis involves setting an arbitrary threshold on what are essentially continua.

It has been customary in work on LI and RD to focus on specific developmental disorders, that is, those where a significant discrepancy exists between language or literacy and general intelligence. However, such

TABLE 8.4. Basic Characteristics of Language Impairment, Reading Disability, and Speech-Sound Disorder

	LI	RD	SSD
Synonyms	• Developmental dysphasia • Developmental language disorder	• Developmental dyslexia	• Phonological disorder • Articulation disorder
Defining characteristics	• Expressive and/or receptive language development is impaired in the context of otherwise normal development (i.e., nonverbal IQ and self-help skills) • Language impairment interferes with activities of daily living and/or academic achievement	• Child has significant difficulty learning to read accurately and fluently despite intelligence within normal limits and adequate opportunity to learn	• Child substitutes or omits sounds from words more than do same-age peers • Speech production errors interfere with intelligibility of speech
Exclusionary criteria	• Severe neglect • Acquired brain damage • Significant hearing impairment • Known syndrome, such as autistic disorder	• Inadequate educational opportunity • Acquired brain damage • Significant hearing impairment • Known syndrome, such as autistic disorder	• Structural or neurological abnormality of articulators • Significant hearing impairment • IQ < 70
Prevalence	• Depends on cutoff used • Epidemiological study (Tomblin et al., 1997): 7.4% (confidence interval 6.3–8.5%) of 6-year-olds met psychometric criterion	• Depends on cutoff used • Typical value is around 9%	• 2–13% (mean = 8.2%) (Shriberg et al., 1999)

(continued)

TABLE 8.4. *(continued)*

	LI	RD	SSD
Odds ratio M:F	• 3 in referred sample (Broomfield & Dodd, 2001); 1.5 in epidemiological sample (Tomblin et al., 1997)	• 1.9 to 3.3 in four epidemiological studies (reviewed by Rutter et al., 2004)	• 1.5 to 2.4 (mean = 1.8) (Shriberg et al., 1999)
Risk factors	• Family history has significant effect • No effect of parental education; slight effect of birth order (later-born at more risk) (Tomblin et al., 1991)	• Parental education • Home literacy environment • Bioenvironmental risk factors, such as lead poisoning and head injuries	• No effect of race, socioeconomic status, or otitis media history, but significant effects of gender, family history, and low maternal education (Campbell et al., 2003)

definitions have been criticized on both logical and practical grounds. In the field of reading disability, it is now broadly accepted that it is not valid to distinguish between children who have a large discrepancy between poor reading and IQ, and those who do not. Both types of poor reader have similar underlying deficits in phonological processing and both respond to similar kinds of treatment (see review in Fletcher, Foorman, Shaywitz, Shaywitz, & Tager-Flusberg, 1999). Analogous arguments have been advanced for LI (e.g., Bishop & Snowling, 2004). Although the focus here is on children of broadly normal nonverbal ability, we use the terms RD and LI without the "specific" prefix rather than requiring a discrepancy-based definition of these disorders.

It is useful to consider cognitive models of LI, RD, and SSD in the context of typical development reviewed earlier, and in relation to each other. The connectionist models in Figures 8.1 and 8.2 demonstrate that a problem in speech production such as that found in SSD could have at least four causes, including (1) a bottom-up problem in processing acoustic features, (2) a motor problem in planning and producing articulatory gestures, (3) a problem learning the mapping between the two, (4) a problem distinguishing which phonetic differences signal differences in meaning and which do not because of weak semantic representations, or some combination of these four problems. Hence, these models suggest that there could be bottom-up auditory, representational (phonology in RD and syntax in LI), top-down semantic, learning, and multiple deficit theories of RD and LI. As we discuss below, existing cognitive models of these disorders have focused on single cognitive deficits and have tended to be static rather than developmental. That is, they have posited a congenital deficit in either a bottom-up auditory skill or a particular kind of representation (phonology or syntax) and have not considered the possibilities of how deficits might emerge from a developmental process or how deficient learning of new mappings between representations could cause disorders.

Language Impairment

A broad distinction can be drawn between two classes of LI models: those that regard the language difficulties as secondary to more general nonlinguistic deficits, and those that postulate a specifically linguistic deficit. The best-known example of the first type of model is the rapid temporal processing (RTP) theory of Tallal and colleagues, which maintains that language learning is handicapped because of poor temporal resolution of perceptual systems. This bottom-up auditory model of LI has also been applied to RD and SSD.

The first evidence for the RTP theory came from a study where children were required to match the order of two tones (Tallal & Piercy, 1973). When tones were rapid or brief, children with LI had problems correctly identifying them, even though they were readily discriminable at slow presentation rates. The theory has continued to develop over the years, and Tallal (2004) proposed a neural basis in the form of spike-timing-dependent learning. Tallal argued that although the underlying mechanism affected all auditory stimuli, its effects were particularly detrimental to language learning because development of neural representations of phonemes depends on fine-grained temporal analysis. Children who have poor temporal resolution will chunk incoming speech in blocks of hundreds of milliseconds rather than tens of milliseconds, and this will affect speech perception and hence aspects of language learning.

Another theoretical account that stresses nonlinguistic temporal processing has been proposed by Miller, Kail, Leonard, and Tomblin (2001), who showed that children with LI had slower reaction times than did control children matched on nonverbal IQ on a range of cognitive tasks, including some, such as mental rotation, that involved no language. Unlike the RTP theory, this account focuses on slowing of cognition rather than perception.

A more specialized theory is the phonological STM deficit account of specific language impairment (SLI) by Gathercole and Baddeley (1990a). These authors noted that many children with SLI are poor at repeating polysyllabic nonwords, a deficit that has been confirmed in many subsequent studies (Graf Estes, Evans, & Else-Quest, 2007). This deficit has been interpreted as indicating a limitation in a phonological STM system that is important for learning new vocabulary (Gathercole & Baddeley, 1990b) and syntax. This theory, like the more specifically linguistic theories discussed later, places the core deficit in a system that is specialized for language processing, but the system is for memory and learning rather than for linguistic representations per se.

More recently, Ullman and Pierpont (2005) proposed a theory that encompasses both STM and syntactic deficits under the umbrella of "procedural learning," which is contrasted with a declarative learning system that is involved in learning new verbal information. They argue that LI is not a specifically linguistic disorder but is rather the consequence of an impaired system that will also affect learning of other procedural operations, such as motor skills.

Many authors, such as Bates (2004), have argued that domain-general deficits in cognitive and perceptual systems are sufficient to account for LI. This position differs radically from linguistic accounts of LI, which maintain that humans have evolved specialized language-learning mechanisms and that LI results when these fail to develop on the normal schedule. Thus, language-specific representational theories of LI coexist with similar linguistic theories of RD and SSD that focus on phonological representations. A range of theories of this type for LI focus on the syntactic difficulties that are a core feature of many children with LI. Children with LI tend to have problems in using verb inflections that mark tense, so they might say "yesterday I walk to school" rather than "yesterday I walked to school." Different linguistic accounts of the specific nature of such problems all maintain that the deficit is located in a domain-specific system that handles syntactic operations and is not a secondary consequence of a more general cognitive processing deficit (see, e.g., Rice & Wexler, 1996; van der Lely, 1994).

Although these various theories of LI focus on different perceptual, cognitive, and linguistic deficits, they are nonetheless hard to choose between for several reasons. First, the theories do not necessarily predict pure deficits in just one area—for instance, the RTP theory predicts that children with SLI will have phonological and syntactic problems, but the theory regards these as secondary to the basic perceptual deficit. Even where a domain-specific linguistic deficit is postulated, it could be argued that other more general deficits may coexist, perhaps because of pleiotropic effects of genes. Second, it is often easy to explain away a failure to find a predicted deficit on the grounds that the child has grown out of the deficit (which nevertheless has affected language acquisition) or that the deficit applies only to a subgroup of children with SLI.

Studies that examine deficits predicted by different theories in the same children aid in disentangling different theoretical accounts. Bishop et al. (1999) studied a sample of twin children, many of whom met criteria for LI. These children were given a battery of tests, including a measure of auditory processing, derived from the RTP theory, and a measure of phonological STM, nonword repetition. Children with LI did worse than controls did on both measures, but some children have normal language despite poor scores on the tests of RTP or nonword repetition. The intercorrelation between the measures, though significant, was low (around 0.3). Furthermore, genetic analysis suggested different etiologies for the auditory deficit, which appeared environmental in origin, and the nonword repetition deficit, which was heritable. One might wonder whether these deficits identify different subgroups of children with LI, but the results indicated that instead, the two deficits interacted such that children with a double deficit were the most severely affected. A similar pattern of results was obtained in a later twin study in which children were assessed on a test of nonword repetition and a test of productive verb morphology (Bishop, 2006). Both measures revealed deficits in children with LI, and in this case, both were heritable, yet the intercorrelation between these measures was low (though significant) and there was no evidence that common genes were implicated. Once again, children with both deficits had the most severe problems, and some children with normal language scored in the impaired range on one of the measures of underlying deficit.

These two studies raise some general points that may also apply to other developmental disorders:

1. Any theory that postulates a single underlying deficit is inadequate to account for the disorder: several distinct deficits seem implicated, none of which is necessary or sufficient on its own for causing LI.
2. Although the different deficits can be dissociated and appear to have distinct etiologies, they tend to co-occur at above-chance levels.
3. It is possible to have a single deficit—for example, in auditory processing or phonological STM—without necessarily showing LI.

Reading Disability

There is greater consensus behind a cognitive model of RD than one for LI. Figure 8.4 depicts the processes involved in extracting meaning from written text. This figure shows that reading comprehension can first be broken down into cognitive components and then into developmental precursors of these cognitive components. One key component is fluent printed word recognition, which is highly predictive of reading comprehension, especially in the early years of reading instruction (Curtis, 1980). The other key component is listening comprehension, that is, oral language comprehension (Hoover & Gough, 1990).

The terms "developmental dyslexia" or "reading disability" have traditionally been reserved for children who have difficulties with basic printed word recognition. It is possible for a child to have reading comprehension problems despite adequate printed word recognition, but this is not counted as dyslexia. Instead, individuals with such problems are described as poor comprehenders, and the cognitive causes of their reading comprehension problems are distinct from those that interfere with word recognition (Nation, 2005).

Printed word recognition can be broken into two component written-language skills, phonological and orthographic coding (Figure 8.4).

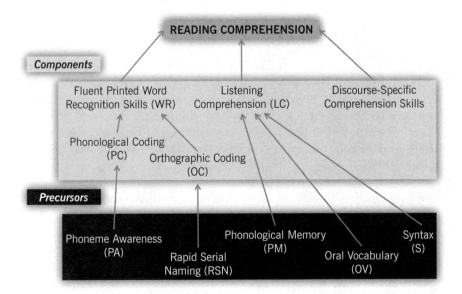

FIGURE 8.4. The processes involved in extracting meaning from written text.

Phonological coding refers to the ability to use knowledge of rule-like letter–sound correspondences to pronounce words that have never been seen before (usually measured by pseudoword reading); orthographic coding refers to the use of word-specific patterns to aid in word recognition and pronunciation. Words that do not follow typical letter–sound correspondences (e.g., *have* or *yacht*) must rely, at least in part, on orthographic coding to be recognized, as do homophones (e.g., *rows* vs. *rose*).

A large body of work has shown that most children with RD have disproportionate problems with pseudoword reading and that this deficit in phonological coding is related to poor phonological awareness. Phonological awareness is measured by tasks that require manipulation of the sound structure of spoken words (e.g., "what is cat without the /k/?"). Despite agreement about the importance of phoneme awareness deficits in RD, there is disagreement about whether these difficulties are themselves caused by lower-level processing deficits. Phoneme awareness is a complex meta-linguistic skill that clearly involves multiple components. One argument is that phoneme awareness deficits arise from impaired phonological representations (Fowler, 1991; Swan & Goswami, 1997a). Another argument postulates that the central deficit is not specific to language, but rather is a consequence of the same RTP deficit proposed as an explanation for SLI (Tallal, 1980). However, evidence for the RTP hypothesis for RD is patchy at best (see McArthur & Bishop, 2001, for a review).

A parsimonious explanation for current data is that deficits in phonological representations lead to both phoneme awareness and phonological coding difficulties in RD. The phonological representations hypothesis is appealing because it helps explain why RD is associated not only with deficits in phoneme awareness, but also with impairments on a wide variety of phonological tasks, including phonological memory (Byrne & Shea, 1979; Shankweiler, Liberman, Mark, Fowler, & Fischer, 1979) and picture naming (Fowler & Swainson, 2004; Swan & Goswami, 1997b).

An important caveat is that the relationship between phoneme awareness and reading is bidirectional, so that over time, poor reading also causes poor phoneme awareness (Morais et al., 1979; Perfetti, Beck, Bell, & Hughes, 1987; Wagner, Torgesen, & Rashotte, 1994). Another caveat is that the evidence for the emergence of phoneme awareness being a necessary precursor for reading development is not airtight (Castles & Coltheart, 2004) because longitudinal studies supporting this claim have not completely eliminated the confound of preschoolers already having some reading skill at time 1. A recent study found that children with chance-level performance on phoneme awareness tasks could nonetheless use letter names to learn letter sounds and thus begin to decode printed words (Treiman, Pennington, Shriberg, & Boada, 2008). So explicit phoneme awareness may not be necessary for learning to read, but it seems clear that appropriately structured phonological representations are needed. The exact meaning of "appropriately structured" is still unclear in the context of reading development. As discussed above, phonological representations develop and can develop atypically in a variety of ways. The nature of the underlying phonological deficit in RD is the subject of several hypotheses, including that children with RD (1) lack segmental phonological representations (Boada & Pennington, 2006; Fowler, 1991), (2) have problems detecting temporally extended, suprasegmental information in phonological representations, the amplitude envelope of an utterance (Goswami et al., 2002), (3) retain very fine grained allophonic representations, which are sound distinctions below the level of the phoneme (Serniclaes, Van Heghe, Mousty, Carre, & Sprenger-Charolles, 2004), or (4) have less distinct phonological representations (Elbro, Borstrom, & Petersen, 1998). More research is needed to test these hypotheses not only in RD, but also across all three disorders considered here. For instance, Corriveau, Pasquini, and Goswami (2007) have recently extended Goswami's suprasegmental theory of RD to LI. These three disorders share deficits on broad phonological measures, such as phonological awareness or nonword repetition, but they can differ in how their phonological representations are deficient.

Because RD is often comorbid with LI, the question is raised as to the extent to which RD is associated with broader language deficits, for example, as measured by tests of vocabulary and syntax. Although the phonological deficit hypothesis stresses children's difficulties in learning letter–sound mappings, poor general language skills could also handicap reading acquisition because one can use linguistic context to infer meaning of a novel word (e.g., Cain, Oakhill, & Lemmon, 2004). On IQ tests, children with RD tend to underperform relative to their typically developing counterparts not only on phonological tasks, such as digit span, but also on all verbal subtests (D'Angiulli & Siegel, 2003). Some of this performance deficit likely results from RD, since children with reading difficulties have impoverished opportunities to learn from print (cf. Scarborough & Parker, 2003; see also Stanovich, 1986), but some may well reflect subtle, wide-ranging language impairments. The evidence on this point from predyslexic children is particularly compelling, because deficits on a wide range of language skills are evident before they learn to read (Pennington & Lefly, 2001; Scarborough, 1990).

The presence of comorbid language problems in RD raises doubts that a phonological deficit is sufficient to cause RD. Moreover, as is discussed below, children with SSD have phonological deficits similar to those found in RD, but they usually do not develop RD unless they have comorbid LI. It appears that normal performance on rapid serial naming (RSN) tasks is a protective factor (Peterson, Pennington, Shriberg, & Boada, 2009; Raitano, Pennington, Tumck, Boada, & Shriberg, 2004). RSN is impaired in both RD and attention-deficit/hyperactivity disorder (ADHD) (Shanahan, Pennington, & Willcutt, 2008), so RSN appears to be a cognitive risk factor shared by RD and ADHD. Moreover, because nonlinguistic processing speed measures such as perceptual speed tasks (Wechsler Symbol Search) played a role similar to that of RSN as a cognitive risk factor for both RD and ADHD, it does not appear that the RSN problem is just a by-product of phonological or name-retrieval problems. My colleagues and I recently tested the hypothesis that processing, speed (sometimes called perceptual speed) is a shared risk factor for RD and ADHD, using structural equation modeling (McGrath et al., 2011). We found that processing speed (i.e., latent traits composed of RSN and nonlinguistic perceptual speed tasks) was a unique predictor of both RD and ADHD symptoms and reduced the correlation between them to a nonsignificant value. Phoneme awareness and language skill were unique predictors of RD symptoms, and inhibition was a unique predictor of ADHD symptoms. These results support a multiple-deficit model of both RD and ADHD. The total variance explained in RD symptoms by phoneme awareness, language skill, and processing speed was more than 80%. Thus, the best current understanding of the neuropsychology of RD indicates that at least three cognitive risk factors are involved, which is consistent with a multiple-deficit model.

At least one of these underlying deficits, deficient phonological representations, overlaps with deficits that are found in studies of LI. However, rather surprisingly, a deficit in RSN is not characteristic of children with LI unless they also have reading impairment (Bishop, McDonald, & Bird, 2009).

Furthermore, although children with RD tend to have lower scores on language tests, they typically do not show the kinds of grammatical limitations seen in LI (Bishop & Snowling, 2004). Overall, multiple underlying deficits appear to exist in RD, as in LI, with the most serious problems being found in children who have two or more of the disorders.

Of particular interest is the indication that at least one underlying deficit, poor phonological processing, is common to both RD and LI.

The procedural learning account of LI is relatively new, and few studies have tested its predictions. Nevertheless, it is noteworthy that it overlaps with the automatization deficit account of dyslexia (Nicolson & Fawcett, 1990). Both theories maintain that specific brain circuitry involving the BG and cerebellum is involved in the poor learning of reading or rule-governed aspects of language, especially phonology and syntax, and in both cases it is argued that associated motor impairments are another symptom of this neurobiological deficit (Nicolson, Fawcett, & Dean, 2001; Ullman & Pierpont, 2005). The automatization deficit account of dyslexia has been challenged as a general account of this disorder by findings that motor impairments are seen in only a subset of cases (e.g., Ramus, 2003). Nevertheless, as we have argued for LI, this does not necessarily mean that these deficits are irrelevant to the causation of the disorder; they may have their effect only when in combination with other deficits.

Speech-Sound Disorder

SSD was originally considered to be a high-level motor problem (in generating oral-motor programs), and children with speech–sound impairments were said to have functional articulation disorder (Bishop, 1997). However, a careful analysis of error patterns rendered a pure motor deficit unlikely as a full explanation for the disorder. For example, children with SSD sometimes produce a sound correctly in one context but incorrectly in another. If children were unable to execute particular motor programs, then we might expect that most of their errors would take the form of phonetic distortions arising from an approximation of that motor program. However, the most common errors in children with SSD are substitutions of phonemes, not distortions (Leonard, 1995). Moreover, a growing body of research demonstrates that individuals with SSD often show deficits on a range of phonological tasks, including speech perception, phoneme awareness, and phonological memory (Bird & Bishop, 1992; Kenney, Barac-Cikoja, Finnengan, Jeffries, & Ludlaw, 2006; Leitao, Hogben, & Fletcher, 1997; Raitano et al., 2004). Though it remains possible that a subgroup of children have SSD primarily because of motor impairments, it now seems likely that the majority of children with SSD have a type of language disorder that primarily affects phonological development. Interestingly, RSN is not impaired in SSD (Raitano et al., 2004), and children with SSD can have persisting phoneme awareness problems but normal reading development (Peterson et al., 2009). Thus, intact RSN appears to be a protective factor in these children.

Evidence for Cognitive Overlap

This brief review of cognitive models of disorders indicates that some close similarities exist in the theories that have been advanced to account for LI, RD, and SSD. For all three disorders, phonological deficits, possibly due to auditory perceptual problems, have been proposed as a core underlying cause. Although this overlap may help explain why the disorders are often comorbid, it leaves us with the puzzle of phenotypic variation between disorders. In short, if the same theoretical account applies to all disorders, why do they involve different behavioral deficits? And why, for instance, do we find children with SSD who have poor phonological skills, yet do not have reading problems? An answer is suggested by our analysis of RD and LI as disorders that involve multiple cognitive deficits. A phonological deficit may be a key feature of all three disorders, yet its specific manifestation will depend on the presence of other deficits. This kind of model is implicit in the analysis by Bishop & Snowling (2004), who argue that LI is not just a more severe form of RD—rather, RD and LI both usually involve poor phonological processing, but LI is seen when this deficit is accompanied by broader difficulties affecting aspects of language such as syntax. The finding (Peterson et al., 2009) that children with SSD often read well despite poor phonological skills indicates that phonological deficit alone will not usually lead to later reading problems—it does so when it is accompanied by poor RSN. A closely similar conclusion was reached (Bishop, McDonald, Bird, & Hayiou-Thomas, 2009) in a study of comorbidity between RD and LI. The study found that children who had LI without RD performed normally on tests of RSN. Both these studies suggest that although phonological deficit is a risk factor for RD, good RSN can act as a protective factor. This evidence for interaction between deficits has implications for how we model comorbidity between disorders (discussed below).

In summary, although cognitive overlap exists among these three disorders (e.g., phonological deficits), the cognitive profile varies as a function of comorbidity. Moreover, these cognitive profile differences appear to map onto the comorbidity patterns reviewed above. That is, the presence or absence of RSN deficits in SSD and LI relates to their comorbidity with later RD. But more systematic research is needed to test how cognitive profiles vary by comorbidity subtype. This research will require large samples that have been followed longitudinally.

CHAPTER SUMMARY

Language processing and development include some components that are specific to language itself (e.g., phonological development) and many that overlap with other domains of cognition. These various cognitive components interact bidirectionally in language processing. Similarly, the brain mechanisms serving language are highly distributed and interactive, and change with development. Thus, the traditional goal of identifying specific acquired aphasic syndromes or developmental language disorders, each affecting distinct aspects of speech and language, and each with a different brain localization, has not succeeded. In contrast, subtypes of both acquired and developmental disorders of language turn out to have considerable overlap with each other.

EXERCISES

1. Watch the video *www.youtube.com/watch?v=jtsfidRq2tw* for a demonstration and explanation of the McGurk effect. (If the video is unavailable, search for a similar video on YouTube.)

2. Using *http://neurosynth.org/locations/0_0_0*, search for "reading" and then "language." Which areas of activity overlap across the two terms? Based on the discussion of multiple and shared cognitive deficits in RD, LI, and SSD, what cognitive processes do you think those active areas support?

CHAPTER 9

■■■■■■■

Disorders of Memory

What sort of life (if any), what sort of world, what sort of self, can be preserved in a man who has lost the greater part of his memory and, with this, his past, and his moorings in time?
——SACKS (1985, p. 22)

A normal healthy person . . . is capable of becoming aware of her own past as well as her own future; she is capable of mental time travel, roaming at will over what has happened as readily as over what might happen.
——ENDEL TULVING (1985, p. 5)

DEFINITION

Our environment constantly changes and we encode some of those changes in our brains in a way that can be demonstrated later behaviorally. So, the term "memory" refers both to a *process* (of encoding or learning information about the environment) and a *product* (the neurally encoded information, often called a "memory trace," that affects later behavior). To be clearer, the process part of memory is often called "learning," and just the product is called memory.

As the two opening quotes indicate, memory, especially memory for events in our lives (episodic memory) is critical to our sense of self. As Tulving's remark suggests, the mechanisms of episodic memory might also be applied to the *future*, allowing us to imagine possible events that have not yet happened. As we will see, one recent development in research on memory is concerned with how possible future events are constructed with some of the same cognitive mechanisms that permit recollection of past events.

Some highlights in the history of research on memory include the following:

1. Lashley's (1929) search for the "engram" in the early 20th century, which is discussed later.
2. Bartlett's (1932) book *Remembering*, which made it clear that the cognitive process of recollection was not a passive process of looking up an unchanging memory in the mental archive or encyclopedia. Instead, Bartlett clarified that recollection is an active reconstruction, much in the same way that perception is an active process of construction. Bartlett's work set the stage for later research on false memories and the idea that the same constructive process may be involved in prediction and imagination.
3. Hebb's (1949) prescient proposal that formation of a long-term memory (LTM) involved the strengthening of synaptic connections in cell assemblies by means of correlated pre- and postsynaptic activity ("cells that fire together wire together"), whereas short-term memory involved a different process of limited duration.
4. The case of H. M. in 1953, discussed in detail later, which provided a candidate structure (the hippocampus and other medial temporal lobe structures) for Hebb's process of forming new LTMs.
5. Bliss and Lømo's (1973) discovery of long-term potentiation (LTP), the physiological basis for Hebb's process of strengthening synapses, in hippocampal slices from a rabbit.
6. Eric Kandel's (e.g., Kandel & Hawkins, 1993) Nobel Prize-winning work on the cellular and molecular mechanisms of classical conditioning in *Aplysia*, a sea snail.

Although some controversies remain, the brain mechanisms of memory have been more thoroughly researched and are better understood than those for any other domain of behavior considered in this book. At this point, there is converging evidence about these brain mechanisms that comes from multiple methods, including human and animal studies, neuroimaging, computational models, and molecular studies. Much of this research has focused on the hippocampus and other medial temporal lobe (MTL) structures because of their role in forming new LTMs by means of LTP.

Learning and memory are examples of brain plasticity, the capacity of the brain to change its structure in response to changes in neural activity. But learning and memory do not encompass all of brain plasticity, much in the same way that learning does not encompass all of development. That is because there are changes in brain structure that are driven by *endogenous* brain activity (spontaneous firing of neurons), whereas learning and memory result from *exogenous* brain activity (dependent on environmental input). As discussed in Chapter 5, there are examples of abnormal plasticity, such as phantom phenomena and synesthesia, which are not considered to be examples of learning and memory, even though they are produced by persisting changes in brain structure and obviously affect behavior. Other such examples of abnormal plasticity might include "kindling" in seizures or mood disorders, which is discussed in a later chapter. In kindling, prior seizures or prior episodes of major depression or mania often lower the threshold for future seizures or episodes by changing the strength of synaptic connections, thus "teaching" the brain to have seizures or episodes of mood disorder. But kindling is not considered as an example of learning because the brain activity involved is mainly endogenous. Similarly, there are examples of normal plasticity in early brain development, such as the formation of eye-specific layers in the LGN of the thalamus in the fetal brain (Shatz, 1992), that also would not fit the definition of learning and memory, because they are driven by endogenous brain activity, in this case activity in the fetal retinas of each eye.

Changes in the strength of connections between neurons are the physical basis of learning and memory (and plasticity more generally). Since, as far as we know, all neurons in the brain are capable of modifying their connections (synapses) with other neurons, every neuron in the brain is capable of learning and memory. In that broad sense, learning and memory are the *least* localized of brain functions. Yet, the neuropsychology of memory individuates multiple memory systems with different localizations. The resolution to this apparent paradox lies in the unique inputs and outputs of different memory circuits and sometimes in the distinct ways these circuits change connection strengths in their synapses. The brain needs different kinds of memory systems: some that learn very slowly, some that learn in a single trial, some that permanently bind different pieces of information together, and some that bind them only transiently.

So, as we will see in the following paragraphs, the isolated term "memory" is not specific enough for a neuroscientist. That is because there are multiple memory systems, each with somewhat different brain mechanisms, developmental trajectories, and pathologies. Laypeople often use some terms for subtypes of memory in a fashion that is *opposite* to how a neuroscientist would use them. For instance, in describing an older person with amnesia, it is common for laypeople to say that the older person has "lost his [or her] short-term memory." Instead, as discussed later, what is lost in amnesia is the ability to form new long-term memories (LTMs), while short-term memory (STM) is usually basically intact.

The broad category of memory (both process and product) can be subdivided by both time course (how long the memory lasts) and by the content of what is learned (Figure 9.1). Very brief memories (lasting milliseconds to seconds) are called **sensory memory**, and are encoded by briefly persisting activity in the sensory cortex (visual or auditory) activated by the input. Visual sensory memory is called **iconic memory** and lasts only 300–500 milliseconds. You can experience an exaggerated form of iconic memory by looking at a bright light and then closing your eyes. Instead of seeing a black field, you still see the after-image of the bright light. Auditory sensory memory is called **echoic memory** and lasts up to 10 seconds. Its duration has been measured by an EEG method called **mismatch negativity (MMN)**, in which an occasional deviant tone occurring in a string of identical standard tones evokes a slightly different EEG waveform. To localize the source of this EEG signal, brain activity in the same task was recorded using magnetoencephalography (MEG), which found the source was in auditory cortex, as expected (Sams, Hari, Rif, & Knuutila, 1993). Sensory memory is preattentive and automatic, an inevitable brief neural trace of prior sensory processing. Because sensory memory is preattentive, it has a large capacity, much larger than the next two forms of memory, both of which require attention and therefore have a limited capacity. Our sensory organs continually register a vast amount of input from the external world, much more than we can consciously perceive and process.

These longer, transient memories are examples of **short-term memory (STM)** or **working memory** and last seconds (without rehearsal), although their duration can be extended for minutes or longer with repeated rehearsal (without interruptions). But if the rehearsal goes on long enough, the memory begins to be encoded into **long-term memory (LTM)**, which is archival rather than transient. We will say more about the distinction between short-term and working memory in the next chapter (Chapter 10) on executive functions (EFs).

LTM is further subdivided by whether the contents are available to consciousness and can thus be *declared* by the individual or not. **Declarative long-term memory** is also called **explicit long-term memory**, and **nondeclarative long-term memory** is also called **implicit long-term memory**. As can be seen in Figure 9.1, examples of implicit LTM include the following: (1) **procedural memory** (e.g., driving a clutch car or serving a tennis ball), which includes statistical learning, as discussed in Chapter 8;

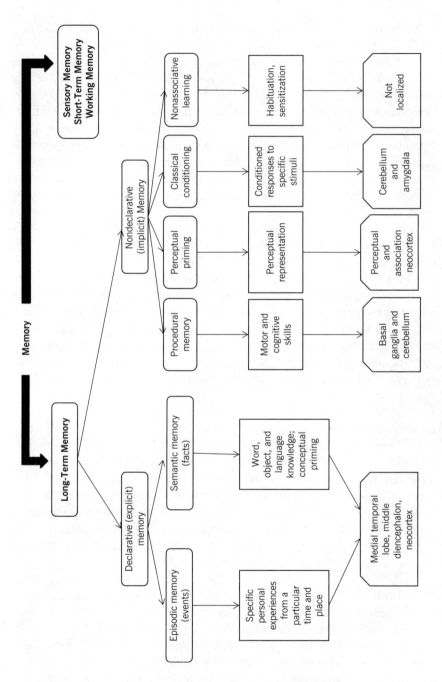

FIGURE 9.1. Multiple memory systems.

(2) **perceptual priming**, in which prior exposure to a perceptual stimulus (e.g., a person's face) facilitates later recognition of the stimulus; (3) **classical** or **Pavlovian conditioning**, in which the repeated pairing of an unconditioned stimulus (e.g., a puff of air to the eye) and a conditioned stimulus (e.g., a blue color patch) eventually leads to the participant blinking his or her eye when only the blue patch is presented; and (4) **nonassociative learning**, which includes phenomena like habituation or sensitization (e.g., no longer being startled by the coffee pot timer every morning). An implicit LTM can be documented by changes in behavior, but the individual may not know he or she has that particular implicit LTM. There are somewhat different neural substrates for each of these forms of implicit memory. For instance, procedural memory is partly mediated by the BG; perceptual priming is mediated by the same parts of posterior neocortex that store perceptual representations; and classical conditioning of the eye-blink response is mediated by the cerebellum, whereas classical conditioning of a fear response is mediated by the amygdala. Habituation and sensitization occur pervasively across animal species and neural circuits, so localizing them depends on what stimuli and responses are involved.

Declarative LTM is divided into two types (Figure 9.1): **episodic long-term memory (LTM)** and **semantic long-term memory (LTM)** (Tulving, 1972). Episodic LTM, the recall of specific events or episodes in one's life, is considered the highest form of memory in evolutionary terms. Semantic LTM is the recall of facts one has learned about the world (but not the particular occasion when one first encountered that fact, which would be an episodic memory). The disorders of memory considered in this chapter are disorders of declarative LTM. We will discuss disorders of procedural LTM in Chapter 10.

As we move from sensory memory to semantic or episodic memory, the representation encoded in memory becomes more abstract, changing from the surface of the input to its gist. We already discussed a similar progression in the chapter on perception. A visual object representation, which is part of semantic memory, has to be fairly abstract to correctly classify all the different sensory presentations of a given object. A similar constructive process must be involved in forming a new episodic or procedural LTM, which is partly constrained by previous LTMs (similar to the consilience constraint in the development of scientific knowledge). So instead of providing a retrospective archive, the biological function of memories is predictive and thus future-oriented. The key evidence for this new function of LTM is contained in Table 9.1 and reviewed in Buckner (2010). New LTMs help organisms make better predictions about how to deal with future events.

So LTMs are dynamic representations that are updated by new memories and reconstructed in light of new world knowledge when recollected, as Bartlett realized (1932). Given all this, false memories are virtually inevitable, and not just an occasional misfiring of the system. The deep subjectivity of memory is a favorite topic in literature, as exemplified by works like the 1950 film *Rashomon* (directed by Akira Kurosawa) and Lawrence Durrell's (1962) *Alexandria Quartet*. In both of these works, the same events are recounted quite differently by each of several different characters.

BRAIN MECHANISMS

Unlike many other functions discussed in this book, memory consolidation has turned out to be surprisingly localized. Why this particular function should be so localized sheds light on the localization debate and sets some limits on recovery of function after brain damage. The MTL is a fairly unique **convergence zone** (Figure 9.2) in the brain that receives inputs from virtually all the rest of the brain, and engages in a distinct form of neural computation.

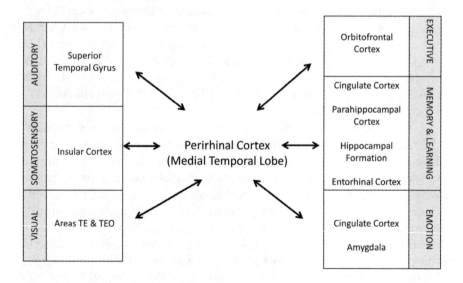

FIGURE 9.2. Medial temporal lobe as a convergence zone. The perirhinal cortex, in the medial temporal lobe, serves as a connectivity hub to visual, auditory, somatosensory, emotional, motor, memory, and executive regions. Based on Murray and Richmond (2001).

The other main part of the brain that is a convergence zone is the prefrontal cortex (PFC), which also engages in a distinct form of neural computation, and which also has distinct limits on recovery of function. But the PFC is much larger, making the MTL, and the hippocampus within it, uniquely vulnerable to injury. Its vulnerability is also attributable to its high level of physiological activity and its consequent vulnerability to decreases in oxygen and glucose supply. In addition, the N-methyl-D-aspartate (NMDA) glutamate receptors in the pyramidal neurons of the CA1 layer of the hippocampus are particularly vulnerable to reduced oxygen (hypoxia). That is because hypoxia leads to excessive glutamate release, and glutamate, an excitatory neurotransmitter, is neurotoxic in large amounts. So, hypoxia leads to differential necrosis (cell death) of pyramidal neurons in the CA1 layer of the hippocampus, and the loss of these neurons causes amnesia because the elements of new LTMs cannot be bound together.

So how does the hippocampus accomplish the function of forming new LTMs? The consensus view is the standard consolidation model. Formation of new explicit LTMs involves rapid binding or learning of arbitrary conjunctions of information, especially across perceptual modalities, such as faces and voices. The MTL, as a convergence zone with unique computational properties, is ideally suited for this kind of learning. Unlike the posterior cortex, which relies on slow learning of overlapping distributed representations (which are subject to interference), the MTL utilizes sparse, pattern-separated representations (O'Reilly & Munakata, 2000). So the MTL performs a unique function of "binding" arbitrary elements of a new explicit memory. This binding function is localized to the MTL, and for episodic LTMs the localization of this binding function may be specific to the hippocampus itself and the CA1 layer within it, as the case of R. B. suggests (Zola-Morgan, Squire, & Amaral, 1986). R. B.'s amnesia was due to a selective loss of CA1 neurons in the hippocampus. But of course this does not mean LTM is *completely* localized to the hippocampus or the CA1 layer within it, since the various structures in Figure 9.2 that project to the MTL also participate in LTM encoding and retrieval. For instance, neuroimaging studies of typical adults highlight the importance of the PFC and parietal lobe in memory encoding and retrieval (see review in Banich & Compton, 2011).

Mechanistically, the binding of arbitrary elements of a new explicit LTM is accomplished through modifications of Hebbian synapses by LTP within the MTL and by signals sent back to the various cortical representations that are being bound. These Hebbian synapses in the hippocampus rely on a particular neurotransmitter receptor, the NMDA receptor.

Blocking NMDA receptors with an antagonist stops the induction of LTP. The discovery of this role of NMDA receptors in LTP has opened up an important window on the molecular biology of LTM, including how genetic variants of these receptors affect memory function. So, signals from the MTL act as "pointers" to the various elements in an explicit LTM. Consolidation of the new LTM occurs gradually over weeks and months as the cortical connections among the various elements become strengthened by correlated firing prompted by these pointer cells. REM sleep is necessary for consolidation and acts as a kind of rehearsal of the new LTM. The model explains amnesia for explicit memories as the loss of the binding function of the MTL. This loss prevents the formation of new explicit LTMs (anterograde amnesia), the loss of some memories that have not been fully consolidated (variable retrograde amnesia), the differential preservation of older memories (temporal gradient in remote memory), and the sparing of memory functions that do not depend on the MTL binding function (procedural LTM, implicit perceptual and semantic memory, STM).

Despite the wide acceptance of the standard consolidation model of how explicit LTMs are formed, there remain important controversies and competing theories (Bird & Burgess, 2008). All these competing theories regard the hippocampus as being critical for episodic memory, but there are key differences in (1) whether they view the hippocampus as having a time-limited role in episodic memory and (2) whether they deem the hippocampus necessary for the acquisition of noncontextual information. The **cognitive-map theory** (O'Keefe & Nadel, 1978) holds that a primary role of the mammalian hippocampus is to construct and store allocentric (world-centered) representations of locations in the environment to aid flexible navigation, for example, from a new starting position. This theory holds that in humans, these predominantly spatial processes have evolved to support the spatio-temporal context of episodic memories. The **declarative theory** (Squire, 1987) holds that the hippocampus, acting in concert with other MTL structures, is crucial for all forms of consciously accessible memory processes (episodic and semantic, recollection and familiarity) for a time-limited period. However, this theory posits that ultimately, all memories are consolidated to neocortical sites and are thus unaffected by subsequent MTL damage. The **multiple memory trace theory** (Nadel, Samsonovich, Ryan, & Moscovitch, 2000), like the declarative theory, holds that the hippocampus, together with other MTL structures, is crucial for the acquisition of episodic and semantic memories. The multiple-trace theory differs from the declarative theory in maintaining that the recollection of episodic memories remains dependent on the hippocampus for the duration of one's life. This theory holds that episodic memories become more resistant to partial damage with repetition and/or rehearsal, whereas semantic memories become independent of the hippocampus and are stored in other brain regions over time. Unlike the previous four theories, the **dual-process theory** (e.g., Vargha-Khadem et al., 1997) holds that the hippocampus is crucial *only* for episodic recollection of the contextual details of an event and that semantic LTMs can be formed *without* a hippocampus, and that familiarity-based recognition processes are subserved by other MTL structures. So, the main points of disagreement among these five theories are 1) whether recall of past episodic memories ever becomes independent of the hippocampus (the declarative theory and the standard consolidation model vs. the multiple-trace theory) and (2) whether semantic LTM requires the hippocampus (the declarative theory vs. dual-process theory).

Another theoretical issue that remains in question is whether all new declarative memories must first be processed in STM or working memory, consistent with the *modal model* of Atkinson and Shiffrin (1968). In other words, is there a unidirectional, serial flow of information from perception to STM to LTM, or could information be processed in parallel such that new LTMs could be formed without passing through STM? Shallice and Warrington (1969) studied a patient with a profound deficit in verbal STM (e.g., on verbal span tasks like digit span) who could still form new verbal LTMs, thus contradicting the modal model. Moreover, hippocampal amnesia patients like H. M. display the opposite profile: intact verbal STM but an inability to form new verbal LTMs. This apparent double dissociation seemed to strongly contradict the modal model, implying that new LTMs could bypass STM. But later research has challenged it because equivalent materials were not used in the STM and LTM tasks, so there was a confound between materials and type of memory (STM vs. LTM). When this confound was removed, the double dissociation was less apparent (Ranganath & Blumenfeld, 2005).

Finally, recent research has uncovered a new function for the hippocampus and other MTL structures, **episodic imagery** (see Table 9.1). As discussed earlier, episodic imagery highlights the predictive value of LTM representations. Memory records the past in a way that is useful for the future behavior of the individual. Tolman (1948) first discovered this predictive value of LTM representations in studies of rats in a maze. He found that past learning in the maze seemed to allow them to construct what he called a "cognitive map" that allowed them to plan future routes that were not previously reinforced. He could not see any way that simple stimulus–response (S-R) connections could explain this novel behavior, so

TABLE 9.1. The Role of the Hippocampus in Prediction and Imagination

Researcher	Discovery
Tolman (1948)	Cognitive maps: rats combine elements of past experiences to guide new behaviors.
Korsakoff (1889); Talland (1965)	These early pioneers in the study of amnesia noted a loss of imagination in their patients, which was also noted in H. M.
Hassabis et al. (2007)	Deficits were reported in hippocampal amnesics during an episodic imagery task.
Schacter et al. (2007, 2008)	(1) Hippocampal activation is present in typical subjects imagining future scenarios. (2) The same cortical system that is active in episodic imagery is also involved in autobiographical memory retrieval.

he postulated that the animal formed a cognitive map or representation that allowed flexible navigation from a new starting place. We can think of this cognitive map as a model or theory of the environment that allows the animal to generate a novel prediction or route to reach a goal from a new starting place.

Clinical observations of patients with explicit amnesia supported this view of LTM in that such patients have a deficit in imagination, that is, they cannot recombine elements of established LTMs to generate an imagined future episode. Subsequent systematic studies of episodic imagery in persons with hippocampal amnesia (Hassabis, Kumaran, Vann, & Maguire, 2007) and neuroimaging studies of typical subjects supported the role of the hippocampus in this important function.

TYPICAL DEVELOPMENT

In this section, we will review when the memory systems discussed earlier become functional in typical development. Additionally, we will consider how these developmental findings constrain neuropsychological theories of memory, including the degree of independence among the multiple memory systems.

In a broad sense, some forms of memory must be present from very early in life; otherwise, *any* development that requires environmental experience could not occur. Because research has documented that infants are prodigious learners in multiple domains, there must be learning and memory mechanisms in place to support this learning. Implicit memory skills could account for much of this infant learning, and in general there is more agreement about the developmental trajectory of implicit memory than explicit memory. Some forms of implicit memory, such as habituation and some types of classical conditioning, are present from birth, while the rest emerge in the first few months of postnatal life. For instance, eye-blink conditioning, described earlier, is evident in the first month of life (Johnson & de Haan, 2011). All forms of implicit memory appear to be fully developed by around the age of 3 years (Johnson & de Haan, 2011), since performance on novel implicit memory tasks does not show subsequent age gains, unlike nearly all the rest of cognitive development. Other evidence bearing on the early development of implicit memory is reviewed in Johnson & de Haan (2011) and includes picture priming (Drummey & Newcombe, 1995), procedural learning in the serial reaction time (RT) task (Thomas & Nelson, 2001), visual expectations (Haith et al., 1988), and statistical learning of pure tone sequences (Saffran, Johnson, Aslin, & Newport, 1999). More work is needed with neuroimaging and other methods to examine how similar the neural substrates of infant and adult implicit memory are.

In contrast, there is controversy about when the explicit memory system becomes functional in early life, but there is fairly good agreement that explicit memory in children requires essentially the same MTL brain structures that underlie explicit memory in adults. This latter conclusion rests on the fact that early MTL lesions in young humans and experimental animals leads to a permanent amnesia, just as it does in adults (de Haan, Mishkin, Baldeweg, & Vargha-Khadem, 2006; Vargha-Khadem et al., 1997). The controversy about when explicit memory "begins" in development shares some of the issues and subtleties that have surrounded other areas of development: what *partial* accomplishments count as instances of the relevant construct, and how much the putative age of acquisition depends on non-memory aspects of the experimental tasks.

Research on the phenomenon of what is called "infantile amnesia" has helped shed light on when the explicit memory system first develops in early life. Infantile amnesia is something we all share: the inability to recall memories of events in our lives much before the age of 3 or 4 years. The explanation for infantile amnesia is a very old question in the history of psychology. One of the earliest explanations of infantile amnesia was provided by Freud, who argued that defensive processes repress these early memories. Although there appears to be an actual phenomenon of posttraumatic amnesia, only a small minority of infants are exposed to early trauma, and even in these infants not all memories are traumatic and need to be defended against. So, Freud's explanation of infantile amnesia has been rejected both on logical grounds and because better explanations have been proposed and tested. Another theory of infantile amnesia is based on the presumed vulnerability of early memories to decay. But considerable research on LTM in typical and amnesic adults has shown just the *opposite*: there is a temporal gradient for remote memories, such that the oldest ones are the least vulnerable to decay. One can see this "first in, last out" process in action in older individuals with amnesia who retain only remote memories and interpret every visitor, including their own child, as being one of their *siblings*. This clinical phenomenon is an example of the rule of Ribot, namely that devolution in old age is development run backwards. So, we can reject this second explanation for infantile amnesia. We now turn to a third, developmental neuropsychological explanation of infantile amnesia, which has been the focus of considerable research and controversy.

Schacter and Moscovitch (1984) and Bachevalier and Mishkin (1984) proposed this third explanation for infantile amnesia: delayed maturation of the MTL systems necessary for explicit memory, with intact early development of implicit memory. Bachevalier and Mishkin (1984) tested this theory in infant monkeys by using two tasks, one thought to be explicit (delayed non-match to sample [DNMS]) and one thought to be implicit (a visual discrimination habit task). In the DNMS task, the young monkey had been previously exposed to one of two objects and had to pick the *novel* object in the pair on a single trial to obtain a reward. This task required recognition memory for the non-novel object based on a single trial and thus required episodic memory, which can be formed from a single episode. In contrast, in the visual discrimination habit task, the monkey was repeatedly exposed to the same 20 pairs of objects, with the same object in each pair always covering a food reward (although the position of the objects within a pair varied randomly). This task required procedural or habit memory, associating a given stimulus in each pair with a motor response that leads to reward. They found a developmental dissociation in performance between the two tasks, with monkeys as young as 3–4 months reaching adult levels of performance on the habit task but not reaching adult levels of performance on the explicit recognition memory task even by 12 months. Similar developmental delays on the DNMS were found in human infants, for whom there was ample evidence of the early emergence of implicit memory as discussed earlier. So, these results supported the delayed maturation of the MTL as an explanation for infantile amnesia.

But later research challenged this hypothesis. One critical finding was that human infants could succeed in a version of the DNMS if the required response was *looking* (i.e., the visual paired comparison task) rather than reaching (Diamond, Werker, & Lalonde, 1994). A similar result was found in infant monkeys. These results suggested that the problem on the standard DNMS was not a lack of explicit memory, but a difficulty with the motor response. This dissociation between looking and reaching performance has been found in many other infant tasks besides DNMS and has been explained by the strength of internal representation needed to guide less versus more mature motor response systems (see Munakata, McClelland, Johnson, & Siegler, 1997). Infant control of eye movements matures much earlier than control of hand movements, so tasks reliant on eye movements could produce earlier evidence of explicit LTM. This result has been found when the task requires learning new faces. Human infants exhibit delayed recognition memory on the visual paired comparison task for specific faces, with a 2-minute delay by a few days of age, and this retention interval increases to 24 hours by 3 months of age (see review in Johnson & de Haan, 2011). So there is evidence of early development of the MTL explicit memory system in human infants.

Further evidence is provided by Rovee-Collier and Cuevas (2009) using their mobile conjugate reinforcement task. In this clever and ecologically valid task, an interesting mobile hanging over the infant moves when the infant kicks his or her leg. (A ribbon connects the infant's leg to the mobile.) Infants learn to move a *particular* mobile when in a *particular* crib by kicking, so this learning is both mobile- and context-specific, thus arguably qualifying as a form of explicit recognition memory. Since there is a linear increase in how long memory is maintained in this paradigm over the first 18 months of life, Rovee-Collier argues for early emergence and continuous development of explicit LTM in infancy. Critics of this view (e.g., Nelson, 1995) argue that the mobile conjugate reinforcement task only taps implicit, procedural memory. However, the results discussed earlier for faces argue against this procedural account of early infant performance in the mobile task. Neuroimaging data may help determine whether the face and mobile tasks engage the MTL in the infant brain. Even though some disagreements remain about the emergence of function of the MTL memory system in infancy, there is enough evidence for its functioning in the first year of life to refute the delayed maturation explanation of infantile amnesia, because infantile amnesia persists until around age 4.

The final and fourth explanation of infantile amnesia is the best-supported one.

> Thus, he was faced with the terror of watching the erasure, day by day, of all his mind had patiently and speechlessly elaborated. The stabbing truth came to him then at once, that when his mind had learned to construct itself in speech images it would be almost impossible to reconstruct its activity during the period when it had had no speech. (Wolfe, 2000, p. 65)

This explanation holds that verbal and other retrieval cues are not available for these infant memories because language and narrative competence have not yet developed. This retrieval deficit theory of infantile amnesia has been tested and supported by Hayne (2004).

DISORDERS

The modern neuroscience of memory begins with the most famous patient in the history of all of neuropsychology, H. M., a Canadian. H. M. developed a seizure disorder beginning in childhood that worsened in his teenage years and was eventually uncontrollable by seizure medications. When he was in his 20s, H. M.'s seizures forced him to quit his job and seek a different treatment. In 1953, when he was 27, H. M. arranged to undergo an experimental treatment for his seizures, bilateral removal of his MTLs (which include the hippocampus, subiculum, entorhinal cortex, perirhinal cortex, and parahippocampal cortex; see Figures 9.3 and 9.4). Because the MTLs also encode olfactory input, the name of some of these structures includes the morpheme "rhinal" based on the Greek name for "nose." At that time, scientists knew seizure activity frequently originated in that part of the brain, but other functions of the MTLs were not well understood. Dr. Henry Scoville, a neurosurgeon at the Hartford Hospital in Connecticut, performed the experimental surgery and documented which brain structures were removed. Although the surgery cured H. M.'s seizure disorder, it left him with a profound problem in forming new LTMs, while leaving older memories much more intact. This dissociation in H. M. between relatively intact established older memories and the inability to form new memories led to the inference that the hippocampus and adjacent MTL structures were crucial for forming new declarative

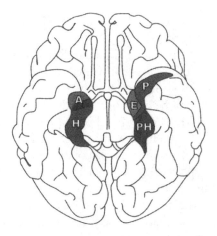

FIGURE 9.3. Hippocampus and related structures. Positions of the amygdala (A), hippocampus (H), entorhinal cortex (E), perirhinal cortex (P), and parahippocampal cortex (PH). From Heilman and Valenstein (2003, p. 521). Copyright 2003 by Oxford University Press. Reprinted by permission.

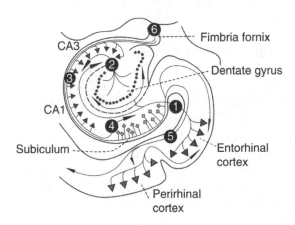

FIGURE 9.4. Internal structure of the hippocampus. Circled numbers represent unique projections within the hippocampal formation. From Heilman and Valenstein (2003, p. 520). Copyright 2003 by Oxford University Press. Reprinted by permission.

LTMs. In contrast to his explicit LTM deficit, H. M. turned out to have intact implicit LTM and intact STM.

H. M. returned to his native Canada after this surgery and generously agreed to be studied by Brenda Milner and her colleagues at McGill University. These studies continued for the next 50 years (H. M. passed away in 2008 at the age of 82) and profoundly changed the neuroscience of memory. Before H. M., the field had been preoccupied with the question of *where* in the brain memories are stored. The famous psychologist Karl Lashley, mentioned in Chapter 3, conducted lesion studies in animals to find where a specific memory or **engram** was stored. He found instead that the storage of an engram was distributed across the animal's brain and that the deficit in a particular memory depended more on the amount of brain removed than on the location of the lesion. He termed this phenomenon **mass effect.** After H. M., memory researchers realized that the crucial question was not *where* memories were stored, but *how* a new memory gets transferred into LTM.

It is worth noting that even after H. M., the field did not immediately settle on this transfer or consolidation interpretation of MTL amnesia. As is usually the case in science, considerable debate ensued and further experiments were conducted to test alternative explanations of this form of amnesia. Some researchers argued that MTL damage produced a retrieval deficit, but this theory could not explain why H. M.'s anterograde amnesia was much worse than his retrograde amnesia. A retrieval deficit alone would predict *equal* severity of anterograde and retrograde amnesia. Subsequent patients with circumscribed lesions of the hippocampus alone exhibited less retrograde amnesia than H. M., but equivalent anterograde amnesia. Moreover, studies of other etiologies of amnesia (e.g., Wernicke–Korsakoff syndrome) in which there is also damage to the PFC found much greater retrieval problems than are found in patients like H. M. Subsequent research has shown a key role for the PFC in memory retrieval. Other researchers argued that hippocampal damage produced an encoding deficit. But that theory could not explain why MTL damage also produced some degree of retrograde amnesia, which affects memories that were already encoded *before* the damage to the hippocampus occurred. So, if the deficit was not in retrieval or encoding, it seemed it must be in the *storage* of the new LTM and that the process of storage must be temporally extended. This storage deficit theory eventually led to the standard consolidation model of how the MTL forms new explicit LTMs. Other etiologies of declarative amnesia are listed in Table 9.2, and most of them affect the MTL.

TABLE 9.2. Etiologies of Amnesia

- Anoxia
- Ischemia
- Closed-head injuries
- Dementias
- Wernicke–Korsakoff syndrome
- Electroconvulsive therapy

An important exception in Table 9.2 is Wernicke–Korsakoff syndrome, also called diencephalic amnesia because the presumed causative damage is to the dorsomedial thalamic nucleus and the mammillary bodies. This damage is produced by a vitamin B (thiamine) deficiency, or beriberi, which can accompany chronic alcoholism. So, interestingly, amnesia can have a dietary cause. Exactly how selective the brain damage produced by thiamine deficiency is or why damage to these particular structures causes amnesia (if it does) remain active areas of research.

There are also disorders that selectively affect implicit LTM, in particular procedural memory, but leave explicit LTM intact. These disorders, which affect the BG, include Parkinson's and Huntington's diseases, which fall in the category of subcortical dementias. In contrast, the most prevalent cortical dementia, Alzheimer's dementia, impairs explicit LTM because of damage to the hippocampus but leaves implicit LTM intact. So there is a double dissociation between explicit and implicit amnesia found in comparisons of these two kinds of dementias. But whether this double dissociation indicates complete independence of explicit and implicit LTM remains controversial because neuroimaging studies of typical adults find some overlapping activation.

CHAPTER SUMMARY

There are multiple memory systems in the human brain, which are mediated by different brain structures, have somewhat different developmental trajectories, and can be selectively impaired by brain damage. Of these multiple memory systems, the most researched is the explicit LTM system, which is subserved by MTL structures, which when damaged lead to a clinical syndrome called amnesia.

EXERCISES

1. Label the following memories as explicit or implicit. What is their subcategory description (e.g., episodic, semantic, procedural, sensory)?

   a. You haven't ridden a bike in 10 years, but when you get on your friend's new bike at his birthday party, it comes right back to you and you have no trouble staying balanced.

   b. A friend is on the phone and asks you to remember an address. She says it aloud to you once and asks you to repeat it back to her about 20 seconds later.

2. In the movie *50 First Dates*, Drew Barrymore's character loses her ability to form new memories after a car crash in which she sustained a traumatic brain injury. What areas of her brain were likely injured? Why couldn't she remember the car crash itself? Why was she able to paint a picture of a boyfriend she met after the crash, despite not remembering his name or who he was? Finally, what would you call this kind of memory disorder?

CHAPTER 10

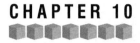

Disorders of Action Selection

[The frontal lobes are] a special workshop of the thinking process.
—BURDACH (1819, cited by Finger, 1994, p. 320)

Luria's position [is] that the frontal lobes contain a system for the programming, regulation and verification of activity.
—SHALLICE (1988, p. 330; on Luria, 1966)

IQ is not lowered by frontal lobe lesions, and may actually be raised.
—KOLB AND WHISHAW (1990, p. 466)

The paradox has been accepted that frontal patients have impaired "planning," "problem-solving," etc. but preserved "intelligence."
—DUNCAN ET AL. (1995, p. 212)

DEFINITION

As the preceding quotes make clear, the PFC has long been regarded as having a special role in aspects of higher cognition, which are now termed "executive functions," "cognitive control" functions, or the term used here, "action selection." But that role has long been a source of controversy (e.g., Goltz, 1888; Hebb, 1945; Munk, 1890). There are several reasons for this long history of controversy about prefrontal functions. Acquired lesions of the PFC are rarer than lesions in posterior cortex, and the clinical symptoms they produce are often more subtle. Patients with prefrontal lesions do not have the dramatic changes in sensory, motor, perceptual, or language functions produced by more posterior lesions. Even some IQ tests do not reveal deficits in patients with prefrontal lesions, especially IQ tests more heavily weighted for crystallized intelligence (acquired knowledge of the sort that is tapped by a measure of vocabulary, for example). Sometimes patients with acquired lesions to the PFC have changes in

153

personality, as observed in the famous case of Phineas Gage (Harlow, 1868/1993), but such changes are not as readily observed or measured as the changes found after posterior lesions. Finally, there have been many fewer studies of prefrontal lesions in experimental animals.

Interest in prefrontal functions was stimulated in the last few decades by the cognitive revolution in psychology and accelerated greatly because of the seminal animal studies of Patricia Goldman-Rakic (1987, 1993) and the advent of neuroimaging. Prefrontal functions have been one of the hottest topics in neuroscience for some time now, and this later research has settled any controversy about the special role of the PFC in typical cognitive functioning and in several prevalent disorders of both adults and children. There are multiple broad terms for the special role of the PFC in cognition, including action selection and executive functions. We will next discuss each of these two constructs.

Action Selection

As described in Pennington (2002), in addition to appraising the adaptive significance of the ever-changing environmental context and generating an appropriate motivational state for that context, an organism must plan and execute actions to deal with that context. Especially in humans, these actions may be directed at a simulated future context and may be in competition with motivations and actions evoked by the immediate context, thus giving rise to the distinctively human virtues of foresight, resisting temptation, and courage. How is action selection mediated by the brain? At a computational level, one of the very difficult problems faced by an action selection system is the so-called "frame" problem. Since the range of an organism's possible actions is infinite, a computational device obviously cannot sort through all of them in real time. How can it narrow the possibilities very quickly to a short, relevant list of alternatives? Humans effortlessly use a representation of the current reference frame or context to do this, but it turns out to be very difficult to program computers to solve the frame problem. As Damasio (1994) and Rolls (1999) have argued, one important input to the human action selection system comes from the motivation system; the motivational state evoked by the current context quickly narrows the field of possible actions. Selection from that much narrower list becomes a tractable computational problem. Anatomically, this must mean there are extensive reciprocal connections between the action selection and motivational systems, and indeed, that is the case. Moreover, some structures in the two systems overlap, since the **orbito-frontal cortex (OFC)** is part of both systems.

There is another important constraint on the action selection system. While humans can think of many possibilities rather quickly, we can generally do only one thing at a time, and to do it properly, some degree of monitoring during the execution of an action is required. Launching competing actions at the same time or launching one during the execution of another will not do. Thus, while the brain is massively parallel, action is relentlessly serial. Step by step we make our way through our lives, mostly doing one thing at a time. This second constraint means that action deselection must work closely with action selection. In other words, inhibition of irrelevant inputs and actions must be an important part of the action selection system. As we will see, there are important inhibitory connections within and between the structures that make up this system.

There are four main interacting brain structures in the action selection system: the PFC, the parietal lobe "how" pathway (described in Chapter 6), the BG, and the cerebellum. The PFC mediates the highest level of planning in the brain (see Figure 10.1), including long-range planning. It receives inputs from the rest of the brain and is thus well positioned anatomically to integrate constraints on action selection. It exerts top-down control over primary and secondary frontal cortex, the

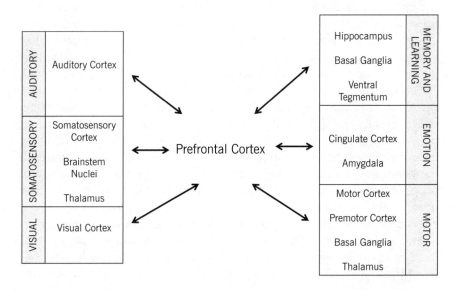

FIGURE 10.1. Prefrontal cortex as a convergence zone. Like the medial temporal lobe, the prefrontal cortex serves as a connectivity hub to visual, auditory, somatosensory, emotional, motor, and memory regions.

BG, and the cerebellum, all of which are more directly tied to motor output. Importantly, it also appears that memories of motor sequences are stored in these other structures; under certain conditions, these automated sequences may actually be implemented as actions without prefrontal input.

Executive Functions

As described in Pennington (2009), "executive functions" (EFs) is an umbrella term for a set of cognitive processes that are important in the control of cognitive processes and action selection, especially in novel contexts or contexts that strongly evoke prepotent but maladaptive responses. EFs are necessary for cognitive flexibility and for controlled or effortful processing. They are mediated by the PFC and closely connected structures like the BG and the anterior cingulate gyrus. Working memory or active memory is a key construct for understanding EFs (O'Reilly & Munakata, 2000). Working memory is a limited-capacity memory system that must be constantly reconfigured (updated) as one solves a problem, and protected from interference by associated but irrelevant information (inhibition). Working memory allows us to generate alternative possibilities and evaluate them, and thus to shift cognitive sets if necessary. So, a list of EFs includes updating, inhibiting, generating, and set shifting.

We can illustrate some of these functions by considering games like bridge and chess. To succeed at these games, one must (1) generate alternative lines of play and look ahead several moves to see where they lead, (2) inhibit prepotent but maladaptive moves, and (3) constantly update the contents of working memory to reflect the current state of the game, which in turn leads to shifting cognitive sets. Practiced bridge and chess players rely on heuristics to reduce the processing demands of play. These heuristics are generally useful tactics, like occupying the center squares of the board in chess or drawing trumps in bridge. But they are not appropriate in every situation. So to perform at a high level of skill, a player must be able to inhibit an overlearned heuristic, shift cognitive sets, and generate novel solutions for the problem at hand. Hence, expert performance in these games requires EFs, even though experts rely on accumulated knowledge to deal quickly with routine situations in each game.

Miyake and colleagues (2000) performed a confirmatory factor analysis of popular EF tasks in the literature, including the Wisconsin Card Sorting Test (WCST), the Tower of Hanoi (TOH), and operation span (OS). They found three distinct but moderately correlated latent traits that correspond conceptually to three of the EFs discussed here: shifting (e.g.,

WCST), inhibiting (e.g., TOH), and updating (e.g., OS). In a later study (Friedman et al., 2006) they tested the relations between these three EF constructs and fluid and crystallized intelligence. They found that updating was strongly related to both intelligence constructs, whereas shifting and inhibiting were not related to either construct. An earlier cognitive analysis of fluid intelligence (Carpenter, Just, & Shell, 1990) also found that working memory capacity was a key contributor to individual differences in fluid intelligence.

While there is broad agreement that the PFC is important for action selection and EFs, there are still competing theories of how different parts of this large and important part of the brain function, and we will return to these competing theories after we review the relevant anatomy.

BRAIN MECHANISMS

In terms of anatomy, the frontal lobes are divided like other neocortical lobes into primary, secondary, and tertiary areas (Figure 10.2).

Primary motor cortex (Brodmann's area 4) is the strip just anterior to the central sulcus in both hemispheres, and like other primary areas exhibits homotopic mapping, in this case to different parts of the body that can be moved voluntarily. This map is called the **motor homunculus**.

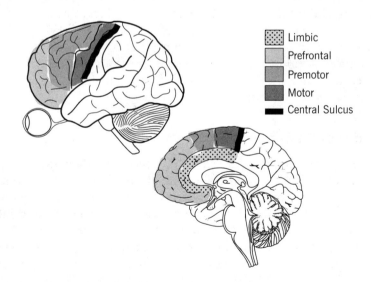

FIGURE 10.2. Lateral and midsagittal views of the frontal lobe areas.

Primary motor cortex projects directly to spinal and facial nerves (and to the BG, as seen in Figure 10.1) and so has direct control over bodily movements. Unilateral lesions in primary motor cortex affect speed and strength of motor movements on the contralateral side of the body, especially fine-motor movements. Secondary motor cortex, also called premotor cortex, includes the supplementary motor area (Brodmann's area 6), the frontal eye fields (Brodmann's area 8), and Broca's area (Brodmann's area 44). Secondary motor cortex is involved in movement planning, especially of sequences of movements, and has reciprocal connections to both primary motor cortex and to the tertiary PFC. Finally, the PFC is divided into lateral (Brodmann's areas 9, 10, and 46), ventral (Brodmann's areas 11, 12, 13, and 14), and medial (Brodmann's areas 25 and 32) areas, which have somewhat different functions as discussed below. All three areas have an active maintenance or working memory function but differ in the content that is held in active memory because of their differing connections to other parts of the brain.

Like the hippocampus and the rest of the MTL (discussed in Chapter 9), the PFC is a convergence zone, with extensive reciprocal connections to all the rest of the brain, including the BG and thalamus, as depicted in Figure 10.1. There are also reciprocal connections between lateral PFC and posterior neocortex that support cognitive working memory and what are called "cool" EFs, in contrast to "hot" EFs, which regulate emotions and motivations, as discussed later. Reciprocal connections between the ventral and medial PFC and the limbic system and various brainstem nuclei support motivational working memory and "hot" EFs, which are important for the integration of action selection and motivation (covered in more detail in Chapter 11). There are also reciprocal connections between the ventral and medial PFC and the anterior insula, which is specialized for self-relevant interoception, like pain.

Theories of Prefrontal Function

As mentioned earlier, there are competing theories of how different parts of the PFC work to accomplish the broad functions of action selection and EFs. Perhaps more than is the case for any other part of the brain, the tension between specialization and integration is fundamental to thinking about prefrontal functions. To understand this point, consider theories of the PFC that divide working memory by content (e.g., spatial, object, and motivational), such as Goldman-Rakic's (1983, 1987) theory or that of Smith and Jonides (1999). Or consider a theory such as Fuster's (1989) or Diamond's (1989) that assigns different processes to different portions of

PFC, such as working memory to dorsolateral PFC (DLPFC) and inhibition to OFC. If PFC functions are specialized according to content or process, then how does the PFC integrate across contents or processes in tasks or real-world situations? If the PFC is a "global workspace" (Duncan, 2001) that accomplishes action selection by integrating all the relevant constraints, then it must be able to integrate across working memory contents, or across working memory and inhibition.

Another key issue faced by theories of PFC functioning is the permanence of the learning that happens in the PFC itself. For instance, one theory of the PFC is that it learns scripts for actions (Grafman, 2002), whereas most other theorists regard the PFC as a buffer for temporary storage of information relevant to the current task. For instance, Miller and colleagues (Freedman, Riesenhuber, Poggio, & Miller, 2001) used single-unit recordings in the lateral PFC of monkeys as they learned to categorize cat versus dog stimuli (which varied continuously from most dog-like to most cat-like, similar to categorical perception tasks discussed in Chapter 8). Because of this stimulus continuum, the monkeys had to learn abstract principles to make the correct categorical judgment. Neurons sensitive to this distinction were found widely distributed over the PFC. The experimenters then taught the same monkeys a different categorization task, discriminating particular pairings of dogs and cats, a task for which the previous learning was irrelevant. Now the same parts of the PFC responded to the new category distinction and not the old one. These results suggest that PFC learning is transient rather than permanent. This transient learning could be accomplished by plasticity in PFC neurons themselves or by gating of different populations of PFC neurons by the BG or some combination of these two mechanisms.

These results are also consistent with an influential theory of PFC functioning proposed by Duncan (2001), called the *adaptive coding model*. This model holds that lateral PFC neurons are highly responsive to current specific task demands and thus are highly flexible across task demands, even though they are not completely equipotential. Some neurons respond preferentially to objects versus locations, for instance, consistent with content-based theories of working memory (e.g., Smith & Jonides, 1999), but both types of neuron increase their firing rate in a task that depends on object information and vice versa. So, the content specializations of these lateral PFC neurons are not absolute and lean toward integration over specialization.

There are nonetheless dimensions of specialization across the PFC. O'Reilly (2010) has integrated these various dimensions of PFC function into his WHACH model (WH = what vs. how, or object vs. spatial representations; A = anterior to posterior gradient; and CH = cold vs. hot EFs). The "what versus how" distinction was discussed in Chapters 6 and 7, on perception and attention. Briefly, the ventral visual pathway is specialized for object representations (i.e., "what"), whereas the dorsal visual pathway is specialized for spatial representations that permit movement planning (i.e., "how"). Each of these visual pathways in the posterior cortices projects to different parts of the lateral PFC, permitting somewhat distinct working memory representations of "what" versus "where" information. So-called "hot" EFs, those involving emotion and personally relevant information, are somewhat localized to the orbital and medial PFC. As already indicated in the section above on the anatomy of the entire frontal cortex, there is also a posterior to anterior abstractness gradient, which reaches the highest level of abstraction in the frontal pole. This abstractness gradient is consistent with hierarchical theories of action selection and cognitive control. Nonetheless, this model is still a unitary model in that interactions among regions of PFC across these three dimensions allow for integration in action selection.

TYPICAL DEVELOPMENT

As described in Pennington (2002), the action selection system, like the motivation system, is an open and developing one, which can be modified by both genetic and environmental influences. The system is open to the environment because actions are nearly always embedded in a social context, which is either immediately present or simulated, so relationships help regulate action selection, either quite directly in young children or more indirectly in older children and adults. Moreover, one of the important functions of a protracted human childhood is to allow for the parental and cultural transmission of patterns of action. Obviously action selection develops, from the infant with little motor control except for eye movements, to the toddler whose attempts at consolidating autonomous action control are evident in the "terrible 2's," to the domination of action selection by peer culture in middle childhood and early adolescence, and hopefully on to the more flexible and long-term patterns of action selection characteristic of adulthood. There are also genetically influenced individual differences in the action selection system, and there are many possibilities for how these genes could work, including receptor characteristics and distributions, learning rates, and connectivity. Dopamine (DA) receptors are denser in the PFC and BG than in other brain regions, so genetic influences on DA receptors could lead to individual differences in action selection. Another important developmental mechanism that genes regulate is increasing structural and functional connectivity between the PFC and the rest of the brain. In sum, just as in the case of the state regulation system discussed in Chapter 11, both genes and environments act on the same developing neural system to produce individual differences in a key psychological process for mental health, action selection.

The development of the structure and functions of the PFC is more protracted than that for any other part of the brain. The role of the PFC as a convergence zone depends on its white matter connections with other brain regions, and some of these white matter connections have a protracted course of development (Plate 10.1 in the color insert). Functional connectivity studies of development going back to Thatcher (1992) show a pattern in which long-range connectivity, such as that between posterior cortex and PFC, increases, and short-range connectivity declines. As the adaptive coding model (Duncan, 2001) of PFC function indicates, the PFC is highly flexible in what information it represents, making it an ideal "executive" for coordinating cognitive development through interaction with other brain structures. In this view, the PFC supervises new learning and then "delegates" learned tasks to posterior cortex, consistent with the interactive specialization theory discussed earlier. So, the PFC should be activated by tasks that are in the child's and adolescent's "proximal zone of development" (Vygotsky, 1979). Which tasks fall into this "zone" at any given time depends on the states of development of other systems that provide input to the PFC. So, for instance, the PFC will exhibit its influence on tasks that require eye movements earlier in development than it will on tasks that require hand movements, due to the developmental sequencing of these motoric responses.

Empirical research on the development of PFC indicates it is active as early as 3–6 months but is not functionally mature until after adolescence. As discussed in Johnson and de Haan (2011), important groundbreaking research on PFC development was conducted by Adele Diamond and Patricia Goldman-Rakic (e.g., Diamond & Goldman-Rakic, 1989) in parallel studies of the development of A-not-B task performance in human and monkey infants (from 7½ to 12 months in human infants and 1½ to 4 months in monkey infants). In the A-not-B task, which is virtually identical to the delayed response task studied in nonhuman primates, the infant is seated in front of two hiding "wells," each covered by a cloth. The experimenter hides an interesting object in well A and lets the infant retrieve it; this sequence is repeated several times. Then the experimenter hides the object in well B, in full view of the infant, and again encourages him or her to retrieve it. Infants of 7½ months of age typically fail by continuing to search in well A (the classic A-not-B error). This persevera-tive behavior is similar to what is observed in monkeys with PFC lesions on the delayed response task and in adult humans with PFC lesions on other tasks (and sometimes even this one). These studies by Diamond and Goldman-Rakic (1989) demonstrated that performance on this Piagetian measure of object permanence exhibited a similar developmental trajec-tory in both species and specifically depended on the integrity of the PFC (as shown by lesion studies in the infant monkeys and corroborated by later EEG studies of human infants). Research on affective decision mak-ing in adolescents using a gambling task (a measure of "hot" EF) showed a protracted development course in both behavior and in brain activity in PFC and its links to striatal reward centers (Crone & Westenberg, 2009).

DISORDERS OF THE PREFRONTAL CORTEX

In this section, we will discuss disorders of the PFC and critically examine how well explained they are. These disorders span all three broad types of behavioral disorders considered in this book: neurological, neurodevelop-mental, and psychiatric. We will begin with neurological disorders, which are defined by their neuropathology. These neurological disorders have provided insights that have helped us understand behaviorally defined dis-orders of EFs.

Neurological Disorders

Clinical neurology (e.g., Filley, 2011) recognizes three somewhat distinct syndromes produced by acquired damage to different parts of the PFC: an orbitofrontal or **ventral syndrome** (also called a pseudopsychopathic syndrome), a **lateral syndrome** (also called a dysexecutive syndrome), and a **medial syndrome** (also called a pseudodepressed syndrome). There are also neurological disorders, such as Parkinson's disease (PD), that mainly affect the BG, which also affect action selection.

The key characteristic of the *orbitofrontal syndrome* is inappropriate social behavior or deportment, including impulsive sexual comments or behaviors, an immature joking attitude (called *Witzelsucht* in German), lack of empathy, and sometimes public incontinence. These symptoms explain why it is also called the pseudopsychopathic syndrome. Psycho-pathy is a form of antisocial personality disorder, whose developmental precursor can be conduct disorder (CD). Patients with these psychiatric disorders violate social and legal norms and have reduced empathy for the suffering of others. Patients with the orbitofrontal syndrome also exhibit very poor decision making and a decreased ability to learn from mistakes, and are often regarded by relatives and friends as having suffered a marked change in personality, as was the case for the classic example of this syndrome, Phineas Gage (Harlow, 1868/1993). Despite these very impairing symptoms, these patients are usually much less impaired on standard neuropsychological tests, including standard tests of "cold" EFs, like the Wisconsin Card Sorting Test (WCST). Several neuropsychological explanations have been offered for these abnormal behaviors, from a general deficit in inhibition (Fuster, 1989) to a more specific deficit in what we might call social–emotional working memory, which is captured by Damasio's (1994) "somatic marker" hypothesis. Somatic markers, according to Damasio, are representations of motivational states and consequences held online in the OFC to guide action selection in social situations, much in the same way cognitive representations are held online in the DLPFC to guide cognitive problem solving ("cold" EFs).

So, partly because of Damasio's work, there is now wide agreement that the OFC mediates "hot" EFs. We all have an intuitive sense of what somatic markers are when we quickly size up a new situation and get a "gut level" response that helps us to quickly decide to approach or avoid it. The OFC can represent such somatic states because of its connectivity to subcortical structures like the amygdala and nucleus accumbens that are important for emotion and motivation. Damasio and colleagues have demonstrated that patients with OFC lesions fail at tasks of affective decision making, like gambling tasks, in which typical individuals quickly learn to avoid choices than can lead to big losses. The classic marker task for the OFC in animal studies is the object reversal task, in which the animal learns which of a pair of objects (or colors) leads to rewards and then has to reverse that preference when the other object is now rewarded. Animals (and humans) with OFC lesions learn normally in the first part of the task but then cannot reverse the learned preference (Rolls, 1999). This deficit in object reversal learning can be explained by Damasio's (1994) somatic marker hypothesis as a failure to use somatic markers to learn from mistakes, but it is less clear how Damasio's theory would explain intact reward learning in the first phase of the object reversal task. In summary, although there are promising hypotheses to explain the orbitofrontal syndrome and the functions of the OFC, considerably more work is needed.

A potential neuropsychological opposite of the orbitofrontal syndrome is provided by the psychiatric condition known as *obsessive–compulsive disorder* (OCD), which is defined by recurrent intrusive thoughts (obsessions), usually about potential harm to oneself or important others, which are relieved by recurrent rituals (compulsions). For instance, a patient with OCD may be obsessed by germs and engage in repetitive hand washing to alleviate this anxiety. In imaging studies, OCD is characterized by overactivity in the orbitofrontal lobes, which apparently help mediate obsessions and compulsions. Overconcern about the possible harmful consequences of one's actions is behaviorally the opposite of psychopathy, in which there is marked underconcern about harming others.

The key symptoms characteristic of the *lateral syndrome* are problems with attention, planning, and other novel-problem-solving behavior. Patients with the lateral syndrome perseverate in applying ineffective strategies and exhibit **environmental dependency**, also called stimulus-bound behavior, or in French, *utilisation* (Lhermitte, 1986). Examples of environmental dependency include a patient (1) immediately drinking a glass of water placed in front of him, even if he is not thirsty, (2) picking up another's pen and writing with it, and (3) when visiting the physician's home, hanging pictures lying on the floor or washing the dishes in the kitchen. In each case, the environment elicits a highly practiced habit that is inappropriate for the current context. Less extreme examples of environmental dependency can be found in typical individuals, especially when they are tired or preoccupied, and are called "capture errors," thus illustrating the continuity between normal and abnormal behavior. William James famously went upstairs to his bedroom to change clothes for dinner, but once he was undressed, he crawled into bed! Tim Shallice (1988, p. 328) reported that he walked into the center of a familiar room and immediately began a pulling movement to turn on the light, momentarily not noticing that the cord was hooked behind a cupboard door.

Patients with the lateral syndrome exhibit deficits on the whole range of "cold" EF tests (Kimberg, D'Esposito, & Farha, 1997), including measures of planning, set shifting (e.g., the Wisconsin Card Sorting Test [WCST]), source memory, fluency, inhibition (e.g., the Stroop task), and self-ordered pointing. At the same time, they perform normally on measures of perception, long-term memory, language, and motor and sensory functions. Although these various cold EF tasks are quite diverse in their surface characteristics, they share a "family resemblance" of requiring working memory to guide action selection and to deselect prepotent but erroneous responses (Kimberg et al., 1997; Roberts & Pennington, 1996). So, selective loss or subtraction of this working memory function provides a good neuropsychological explanation of the lateral syndrome, and this explanation is supported by the extensive research on the functions of the DLPFC reviewed earlier.

Of these three PFC syndromes, the medial syndrome is probably the least well understood. The key symptom in this syndrome is apathy, as patients with this syndrome exhibit little spontaneous behavior, hence the designation "pseudodepressed." There is a continuum of diminished motivation in patients with the medial syndrome that runs from apathy to abulia (literally "lack of will") to akinetic mutism, in which there is a complete absence of movement or speech, even though the patient is conscious. Oliver Sacks's (1973) book *Awakenings* provides fascinating case descriptions of akinetic mutism secondary to postencephalitis lethargica, a severe variant of PD. Damage outside the PFC in the secondary motor area, which has a medial aspect, can produce a similar behavioral syndrome. An important lesion site within the medial PFC contributing to this syndrome is the anterior cingulate gyrus (ACG). The ACG has a known role in action and error monitoring, but the theoretical link to the paucity of action observed in the medial syndrome has not been elaborated.

We now turn to a neurological disorder of the BG that affects EFs, namely, PD. PD is a common (1 per 1,000 in the population, with a rate of 1.6 per 1,000 in those over 65 years of age), usually idiopathic (of unknown cause), neurological disease in which characteristic pathology is a loss of pigmented cells, mainly in the substantia nigra (SN), a brainstem nucleus that sends dopaminergic projections to the BG. As will be described later, the DA depletion in PD would reduce activity in the Go pathway in the BG, making it harder to select and execute an action. Hence DA depletion in PD leads to a motor disorder characterized by a resting tremor and rigidity, and by difficulty in the initiation (called hypokinesia) and reductions in the speed (called bradykinesia) of motor movements. Because of these problems in motor initiation and speed, PD patients cannot make the small frequent adjustments necessary for postural stability and so have balance problems. In addition to these motor symptoms of PD, there are characteristic cognitive disturbances, including deficits in EFs and probabilistic learning. In particular, unmedicated patients with PD have diminished reward learning and those medicated with L-*dopa*, a DA agonist, have diminished punishment learning. In fact, medicated patients with PD have an increased rate of addictive gambling, somewhat reminiscent of patients with the orbitofrontal syndrome described above.

To explain this puzzling opposite profile of probabilistic learning in unmedicated versus medicated PD, Frank, Seeberger, and O'Reilly (2004) developed a neural network model of the BG circuits involved in probabilistic learning. This system learns from experience about which actions lead to rewards and which to punishments, and these memories are stored in procedural LTM. As discussed earlier, memory in the PFC itself needs to be transient, not permanent, so the "mental workspace" or rapid access memory (RAM) provided by the PFC remains flexible to deal with new tasks. So, this procedural learning from incentives takes place in the striatum by means of phasic changes in DA released by the SN. Actions that lead to unexpected rewards cause phasic bursts of DA release into the striatum, and actions that lead to punishment cause phasic dips in DA release.

These phasic changes in DA act on two different parts of the striatum, with each part participating in two unique circuits involved in action selection, one that permits an action to be selected and executed (the "direct" Go pathway) and another that inhibits actions the rest of the time (the "indirect" NoGo pathway; see Plate 10.2 in the color insert). The baseline state of this system for action selection is for the NoGo pathway to override the Go pathway; ordinarily, the "brakes" should be on in order to avoid launching extraneous actions that would be maladaptive. Recall, as discussed earlier, that action is relentlessly serial, so the action selection system must launch only one action at a time. The NoGo pathway acts as the brake on the PFC; this pathway consists of the internal segment of the globus pallidus (GPi), which inhibits the thalamus, which would otherwise activate the PFC to produce an action. In this model, the PFC is holding a candidate action on line, but only after the direct pathway inhibits the GPi's inhibition of the thalamus can the brakes be released and action execution occur.

These two pathways are somewhat confusing to understand at first, because *both* pathways from the striatum to the PFC are actually indirect. The direct Go pathway just has fewer way stations (two vs. three), making it *more* direct. Another source of confusion is that to calculate the net effect of a DA burst or dip on action selection in the PFC, one has to multiply the signs of the intervening synapses at each way station. In the Go circuit, a DA burst in the striatum increases its inhibition of the GPi, thereby decreasing the GPi's inhibition of the thalamus (thus taking off the brakes). In the NoGo circuit, there is an extra way station, the external segment of the globus pallidus (GPe). In the resting state, the NoGo portion of the striatum inhibits the GPe, thereby decreasing its inhibition of the GPi, and thus increasing the inhibition of the thalamus (putting on the brakes).

So, the motor symptoms of PD arise because the brakes are on too much of the time, and it is much harder to release the brakes on action selection than it is in individuals without PD. Thus, PD is an example of *horizontal imbalance*, one of the neuropsychological explanations discussed in Chapter 5. In horizontal imbalance, there are two structures at the same level in the brain's processing hierarchy with opposite effects on behavior. Their competition is balanced in typical behavior, but imbalanced in a disorder.

This imbalance in PD has cognitive effects as well as motor effects, and the purpose of the Frank et al. (2004) study was to explore these cognitive effects in the domain of procedural memory. The authors examined performance of medicated and unmedicated patients with PD and controls, as well as performance of a computational model of the BG, on two different learning tasks. One learning task was probabilistic while the second was deterministic. On each trial in both tasks, participants chose one of a pair of two abstract designs (Japanese hiragana characters) and then received feedback about whether their choice was correct or incorrect. In the probabilistic task, this feedback was correct 80% of the time in one pair, 70% in another, and 60% in the last pair, allowing the strength of learning to vary across the six items, and permitting a test of transfer of learning using novel pairs of items. As expected based on previous studies and the DA deficit in PD, unmedicated PD patients performed worse at reward learning than controls, since both tonic and phasic DA depletion suppresses the Go pathway. One *novel* prediction from the computational model was that unmedicated patients with PD would perform better on punishment learning than they would on reward learning. This prediction was confirmed on both learning tasks. The other novel prediction was that medicated patients with PD would show the opposite profile: they would perform worse on punishment learning than they would on reward learning. This second prediction was also confirmed on both tasks.

In sum, PD is a well-explained disorder at the levels of brain, neuropsychology, and behavior, and it best fits a horizontal imbalance model. This work on PD has proven useful in helping to explain two neurodevelopmental disorders: Tourette syndrome (TS) and attention-deficit/hyperactivity disorder (ADHD). As will be explained next, TS is virtually the neuropsychological opposite of PD. ADHD is more complex and is a partial opposite of PD.

Tourette Syndrome and ADHD

Similar to PD, both TS and ADHD, which are neurodevelopmental disorders, have alterations in DA transmission that affect action selection. In TS, children develop chronic motor tics (e.g., eye blinks) and vocal tics (e.g., coughs, grunts, or even swear words, called *coprolalia*). In ADHD, children have deficits in either attention or movement/impulse control (or both). Both TS and ADHD are neuropsychological *opposites* of PD because in each syndrome, the brakes on action selection have been released, leading to nonadaptive actions. But TS and ADHD have important differences and to understand those differences, it is useful to know about the distribution of DA receptors in the brain.

In general, there are two families of DA receptors: D1-like (D1 and D5) and D2-like (D2, D3, and D4). D1-like receptors activate adenylate cyclase and increase cAMP, whereas D2-like receptors do the opposite. The distribution of DA receptors varies across the brain (all five types are found in the cerebral cortex and limbic system; only D1 and D2 are found in the BG; and only D3 and D5 are found in the hypothalamus). D1 receptors are by far the most numerous in the brain. Roughly speaking, D1 receptors are more related to cognition and D2 receptors are more related to motor control, although both D1 and D2 receptors are both related to working memory updating and D1 receptors are also found in the BG. This broad contrast between D1 and D2 receptors is relevant for understanding TS versus ADHD.

TS appears to result from either a shortage of inhibitory striatal spiny neurons or excess striatal DA (Albin & Mink, 2006), either of which would facilitate the Go pathway in Plate 10.2, thus taking off the brakes on action selection and resulting in motor and vocal tics. TS is treated by DA antagonists that act in the BG, possibly on D2 receptors, to increase activity in the NoGo pathway in Plate 10.2, thus inhibiting tics. In sum, TS appears to be primarily a "bottom-up" disorder, but some PFC changes are also found in TS, so that determining which brain changes came first is a challenge.

In contrast to TS, the location of the DA disturbance in ADHD is less clear. Based on extensive animal work, Berridge and Devilbiss (2011) have found that D1 receptors in the PFC are one main target of low doses of psychostimulants (e.g., methylphenidate, which is sold as Ritalin), which calm behavior and enhance cognition. At these low doses, psychostimulants produce somewhat localized increases in both DA and norepinephrine in the PFC. At higher doses, psychostimulants (think recreational doses of meth and cocaine) are behaviorally activating and increase DA and norepinephrine throughout the brain.

Complicating this PFC account of ADHD is the fact that Volkow, Fowler, Ding, Wang, and Gatley (1999) found more binding of methylphenidate in the BG than in the PFC. Methylphenidate is a DA reuptake inhibitor that is thought to act on the DA transporter, which has a dense distribution in the BG compared to a sparse distribution in the PFC. Volkow and colleagues reported that individuals with more DA receptors in the BG find methylphenidate unpleasant (too activating), while those with fewer receptors find it pleasant (Volkow et al., 1999). This pattern of responding to methylphenidate is consistent with an inverted U-shape function of drug response. Consistent with this BG view of ADHD is the fact that ADHD is associated with alleleic variants of the DA transporter (DAT1) gene. In sum, existing studies do not converge on the localization of either the DA deficit in ADHD or the site of action of methylphenidate, and it is possible that *both* the PFC and BG are involved.

Procedural Learning in TS and ADHD

Procedural learning is tapped by motor skill learning (e.g., pursuit rotor and mirror tracing), weight biasing, and prism adaptation, as well as the probabilistic learning tasks used in the Frank et al. (2004) paper. Marsh and colleagues (2005, 2004) found that probabilistic learning was impaired in individuals with TS who were off medication, but procedural learning was intact, as was declarative memory. Marsh et al. (2004) did not examine go learning and no-go learning separately. Palminteri et al. (2009) compared patients with TS and those with PD on a probabilistic learning task both on and off DA medication. This experiment allowed a direct test of the hypothesis that TS is the neuropsychological *opposite* of PD. Consistent with this hypothesis, they found that the patients with TS who were *off* medication were impaired at *no-go* learning but intact on go learning, whereas those with PD who were off medication had the opposite profile, as previously found by Frank et al. (2004). When they were on their usual DA agonist medications, the profile of each group was reversed (Figure 10.3).

GO LEARNING \ NO-GO LEARNING	Less	Equal	More
Less	**ADHD off**		
Equal	PD on ADHD on	**Typicals**	**PD off** TS on
More		PD on **TS off**	

FIGURE 10.3. Reinforcement learning performance for three disorders on and off dopamine medication.

The results for ADHD on various BG-dependent tasks are less clear-cut than they are for TS and PD. Colvin, Yeates, Enrile, and Coury (2003) found that motor skill procedural learning was intact in ADHD. Barnes, Howard, Howard, Kenealy, and Vaidya (2010) found a different implicit learning deficit in ADHD on a serial reaction time task , but not a deficit on an implicit, hippocampally dependent spatial context learning task. They did not report medication status.

Frank, Santamaria, O'Reilly, and Willcutt (2007) used their PD computational model to test its applicability to children with ADHD on and off stimulant medications. It is known that unmedicated individuals with ADHD have low striatal DA levels, which the computational model predicts should produce impaired go (reward) learning and, secondarily, impaired working memory updating in the PFC. Consistent with the model's predictions, unmedicated adults with ADHD had deficits relative to controls in both go learning (on the previously described probabilistic learning task) and in working memory updating on a continuous performance task (CPT); also as predicted, these deficits were eliminated by stimulant medication. These are exciting results because they provide evidence that both motivational (reward learning) and cognitive (working memory updating) deficits in ADHD are caused by low striatal DA. There were also behavioral results that the model did not explain. The unmedicated ADHD group was also impaired in NoGo learning, and these researchers did not find medication effects on another well-documented aspect of ADHD, increased variability in reaction time. They hypothesized that this feature was related to low levels of norepinephrine in the neocortex.

In sum, the neuropsychological explanation of ADHD is less complete and likely more complicated than those for TS and PD. TS and PD are neuropsychological opposites, each involving a horizontal imbalance in probabilistic learning mediated by the BG, which can be partly corrected by medications that alter DA levels. ADHD appears to have both PFC and BG components and involves both DA and NE neurotransmitter imbalances. So, ADHD involves *multiple* cognitive deficits (McGrath et al., 2011) including deficits in PFC-mediated inhibition, norepinephrine-mediated variability in reaction time (greater standard deviation of reaction time), and processing speed (the neural basis for which is less well understood).

Schizophrenia

This disorder typically includes both positive symptoms (e.g., hallucinations and delusions) and negative ones (e.g., flat affect, poverty of speech, and avolition). Providing a neuropsychological explanation for *both* kinds of symptoms has been challenging. Patients with schizophrenia are impaired on various measures of EFs, such as working memory tasks, and have reduced activation of the DLPFC, both at rest and during cognitive tasks. These EF deficits provide a good explanation of the poor adaptive behavior exhibited by individuals with schizophrenia and for some of their negative symptoms. But these EF deficits by themselves do not account for the positive symptoms found in persons with schizophrenia, since patients with many other clinical disorders have EF deficits without having hallucinations and delusions.

One of the best-supported neuropsychological explanations for the positive symptoms in schizophrenia is a deficit in *self-monitoring*, or *action monitoring* (Blakemore & Frith, 2003; Frith, 1987; Frith & Done, 1989). The careful reader will have noted that the medial frontal syndrome, described earlier, has some similarities to schizophrenia. The negative symptoms in schizophrenia are reminiscent of the paucity of behavior found in the medial syndrome (apathy and abulia). In addition, patients with that syndrome also exhibit deficits in action monitoring. So, let us explain what action monitoring is and how it might explain the positive symptoms in schizophrenia.

Going all the way back to von Helmholtz (1867) in the 19th century, psychologists have noted that humans and other animals must distinguish differences in perception caused by their own movements from those caused by changes in the external world. We do not think the world moves every time we turn our head, and it would be very maladaptive if we did. How does the brain make this distinction, which requires action monitoring? Sperry (1950), a Nobel prize–winning neuropsychologist, proposed the concept of **corollary discharge** to explain how the brain is able to discount changes in perception that are produced by the organism's own movements. In his view, when the frontal lobes select and execute an action, they send a copy of that command (called an **efference copy** by Von Holst, 1954) to perceptual centers so they can compensate for the self-produced change in sensory input. Typical humans and other animals do this automatically. The neural circuitry for some forms of this process, such as the **vestibular ocular reflex**, which corrects for perceptual changes caused by the individual's own eye movements, has been thoroughly explored. At a higher level, action monitoring is needed to attribute accurately the source of intentions and other thoughts, which are also "actions" generated by the frontal lobes.

An examination of the hallucinations and delusions found in schizophrenia shows that they are at a high cognitive level and of a particular kind that a deficit in self-monitoring could produce. As explained by Jeannerod et al. (2003), these delusions and hallucinations involve misattribution of the source of actions and thoughts, either underattributions (attributing one's own thoughts or actions to an outside agent) or overattributions (attributing another's thoughts or actions to oneself). These misattributions are examples of what Schneider (1959) called first-rank features of schizophrenia, which he considered necessary for the diagnosis. First-rank features include the following underattributions: (1) auditory hallucinations of hearing voices directed at the self, (2) thought insertion in which an outside agent plants thoughts in the patient's mind, and (3) passivity experiences or delusions of alien control. First-rank features also include an overattribution called thought broadcasting, in which the patient believes another person is uttering his or her own thoughts. In contrast to these kinds of hallucinations found in schizophrenia, the hallucinations caused by other abnormal brain conditions are usually at a lower, perceptual level, such as the vivid visual hallucinations produced by high fevers or by taking LSD or peyote (Tekin & Cummings, 2003).

Behavioral evidence supporting the self-monitoring theory of the positive symptoms in schizophrenia includes deficits in (1) movement correction without visual feedback (Frith & Done, 1989); (2) discrimination of self versus other tactile stimulation (Blakemore & Frith, 2003); and (3) correct attribution of hand movements seen in a mirror to self versus experimenter (Jeannerod et al., 2003). In each paradigm, patients with schizophrenia who had Schneiderian symptoms performed worse than controls or than patients with schizophrenia without such symptoms.

This theory is also supported by functional and structural neuroimaging studies of the ACG in schizophrenia. The ACG lies on the medial surface just beneath the PFC. EEG and fMRI studies confirm its role in error monitoring. For instance, the ACG is the source of a distinct EEG signal, known as error-related negativity (ERN). Patients with schizophrenia do not show normal ERN responses to their own errors (Mathalon et al., 2002), and a similar result has been found with fMRI (Kerns et al., 2005; Nordahl et al., 2001). Structural MRI studies have found reduced volumes in the ACG in schizophrenia (Choi et al., 2005; Wang et al., 2007), consistent with earlier postmortem findings reported by Benes (1993).

CHAPTER SUMMARY

Deficits in various executive functions mediated by the PFC are found across all three kinds of behavioral disorders covered in this book: neurological (e.g., PD), psychiatric (e.g., schizophrenia), and neurodevelopmental

TABLE 10.1. Action Selection Disorders

	Overactive	Underactive
Basal ganglia	TS	PD
Ventral PFC	OCD	CD
Lateral PFC	?	ADHD
Medial PFC	?	Schizophrenia

Note. ?, no known disorder.

(e.g., TS and ADHD). They are also implicated in most disorders of emotion regulation, which are the topic of the next chapter. Progress in understanding how the PFC and closely related structures, like the BG, work together in action selection and deselection has led to major advances in our understanding of most disorders in psychiatry. This progress has been greatly facilitated by (1) neuroimaging studies of PFC structures and functions in typical and atypical populations and (2) neural network models of the PFC and BG. Table 10.1 provides a simple summary of action selection disorders organized by structure (BG and ventral, lateral, or medial PFC) and activity level (over- vs. underactive).

EXERCISE

1. Michael Shermer, executive director of the Skeptics Society and publisher of *Skeptic* magazine, discusses dopamine's role in believing the unbelievable in his TED talk, "The Pattern Behind Self-Deception." Search for it or locate it at *www.ted.com/talks/michael_shermer_the_pattern_behind_self_deception.html*. How does this relate to the positive symptoms of schizophrenia?

CHAPTER 11

■■■■■■■

Disorders of State Regulation

Here in this well concealed spot, almost to be covered with a thumb nail, lies the very mainspring of primitive existence— vegetative, emotional, reproductive—on which, with more or less success, man has come to superimpose a cortex of inhibitions.
— CUSHING (1929, quoted in Card, Swanson, & Moore, 2008, p. 795)

The sylvian fissure is one of the chief boundaries between neurology and psychiatry.
— GIBBS & GIBBS (1948, quoted in Filley, 2011, p. 134)

DEFINITION

In this chapter we come to disorders that have traditionally fallen into the realm of psychiatry and are often not covered in neuropsychology and cognitive neuroscience texts. But the rapidly growing fields of social and affective neuroscience have led to a much better understanding of disorders in these domains. The boundaries among the clinical fields of neurology, psychiatry, and neuropsychology are blurring. In terms of basic science, psychology departments now include cognitive neuroscientists who are actively collaborating with social and affective neuroscientists to the considerable benefit of both fields, and, of course, to the benefit of the three clinical fields just mentioned.

It is increasingly apparent that we should not split social, emotional, and other motivational processes from cognitive functions in our analysis of brain functions. Our cognitive functions evolved because they contributed to basic biological goals: survival and reproductive success. In addition, cognitive processing in the individual is always affected by the individual's current motivational state and is in the service of goals that derive, however circuitously, from social and emotional needs.

We share many social and motivational abilities with other animals, some with virtually all animals (recognition of and preference for conspecifics), others with many other animals (recognition of individual conspecifics), some only with vertebrates (a hypothalamus and peripheral autonomic nervous system to direct basic survival-related behaviors), others with all mammals (attachment, maternal behavior, and pair bonding), and some only with highly social mammals, like wolves, cetaceans (whales and dolphins), and some other primates (play, dominance hierarchies, emotion perception and production, communication, and some degree of imitation). Only a very few social abilities appear to be uniquely human, such as joint attention, theory of mind, extensive use of imitation, and language, whereas our motivational abilities or states are widely shared with other species.

This chapter will focus only on the social, emotional, and other motivational processes that are involved in disorders of state regulation (i.e., mood, anxiety, and addictive disorders) and social cognition (mainly autism spectrum disorder). Though many puzzles remain, we are much closer to neuropsychological explanations of mood, anxiety, and addictive disorders. Even autism, the most puzzling disorder covered in this book, is yielding its secrets to the concerted efforts of neuroscientists working across several levels of analysis. I will first discuss the typical functions (which fall under the broad label of state regulation) that are disrupted in mood, anxiety, and addictive disorders, and then discuss social cognition in the section on development.

BRAIN MECHANISMS

The reader may wonder why I used the term "state regulation" instead of the more usual term "emotion regulation." The reason is that, at the level of the brain, the mechanisms that regulate emotions have much in common with the mechanisms for regulating other motivational states, like pain, hunger, and so on. As discussed in Damasio (2010) and Panksepp and Biven (2012), these basic motivational states are "primordial feelings" in Damasio's terms or "homeostatic affects" in Panksepp and Biven's terms. In Table 11.1 (on p. 183) Below I present a hierarchical brain model of state regulation that includes these other motivational states. To understand these motivational states, we have to look first at much older parts of the brain in evolutionary terms and their relation to the **peripheral**

autonomic nervous system (pANS) outside of the central nervous system (CNS), which is composed of the brain and the spinal cord. From an evolutionary perspective, it is ironic that human neuropsychology is mainly focused on the neocortex, the most recently evolved part of the brain, since its evolution would not have happened if it did not serve basic survival goals still mediated in part by these much older parts of the brain. This bias in human neuropsychology could be seen as a vestige of mind–body dualism, with the supposedly unique human mind deserving much more attention than the bodily functions we share with other animals. In contrast, animal neuropsychology has tended to progress in the opposite direction, from lower functions to higher ones. A mouse neuropsychologist I once worked with, Linda Crnic, told me that in her field the joke was that the neocortex evolved "to keep the dust off the hypothalamus." The hypothalamus is the "well-concealed spot" referred to in the opening quote by Harvey Cushing, a neurosurgeon who was one of the founders of endocrinology, and for whom Cushing's syndrome (characterized by excess secretion of the stress hormone cortisol by the adrenal gland) is named.

The **hypothalamus** and related structures in the CNS allow the "mind" to talk with the "body" and vice versa, so they help solve the mediation problem posed by dualistic theories like that of Descartes. The mediation problem is simply the problem of how an immaterial mind can interact with a physical body. Descartes speculated that the pineal gland performed this mediation function, but he should have picked the hypothalamus. Although modern neuroscience has rejected dualism, it still has to account for how cognitive representations and processes can affect bodily states (e.g., how certain thoughts or words can make us blush) and vice versa (e.g., how a pain or itch in the body immediately focuses attention on that body part). The hypothalamus and its connections to the pANS help explain this bidirectional link between cognition and bodily states, and they play a key role in the model of state regulation presented next.

In this hierarchical brain model of state regulation, "state" means motivational state, of which emotions are a subset. Motivational states include homeostatic drives like pain, hunger, thirst, sexual desire, elimination, and being too cold or too hot, as well as addictive cravings. All these states are represented at multiple levels in the nervous system, some implicit and unconscious and some conscious (Table 11.1), and can arise because of input from the pANS (pain, hunger, thirst, etc.). There are bidirectional connections (both excitatory and inhibitory) between levels, as well as inhibitory connections between opposite valences at a given level. So a state can potentially arise at any level of the system, including in the body, but it then propagates to all levels until an action is taken to terminate the state and return the system to homeostasis. Fortunately, our ANS takes care of many states automatically, without deliberate action on our part and often without consciousness. For instance, we do not decide to perspire or shiver when hot or cold. But we may become conscious of being hot and perspiring or being cold and shivering, and that awareness may lead to a voluntary action to help us return to homeostasis. In this example, the motivational state arose in the periphery and then propagated all the way up to the level of conscious cognitive control or action selection. Because states propagate, they organize and direct various cognitive processes, including attention, perception, motor planning, and both memory retrieval and encoding. Because these states are related to basic survival goals of the organism, they usually have a higher priority than states based on derived goals (e.g., curiosity), as Maslow (1943) recognized in his hierarchical model of goal states. We cannot decide not to breathe, and we cannot effectively pursue derived goals when basic motivational states are highly activated. Pain, hunger, fear, and thirst will trump the pursuit of other goals virtually every time. These motivational states organize the activity of the whole brain in the same way that the cognitive state of attention does (see Chapter 7), and the focus of attention is subordinate to these motivational states when they are activated.

As said earlier, in typical functioning, a state arises and is then satisfied, allowing the system to return to homeostasis. In disorders of state regulation, as will be explained later, states and resulting cognitive processes are exaggerated and often prolonged, and it becomes much harder for the system to return to homeostasis. Although we do not completely understand why an organism comes to have an exaggerated and prolonged motivational state, we do know that emotional conditioning, including fear conditioning, is a very important contributor. Ancient organisms that did not learn to avoid a threat to their life did not survive (Ohman, 2000), so fear conditioning was selected for more than it was selected against. As will be discussed later, this evolutionary theory helps explain the high prevalence of disorders in which negative emotions are exaggerated (depression and anxiety disorders), relative to the prevalence of disorders in which positive emotions are exaggerated (mania).

Now I will discuss the six levels of this model in more detail, beginning at the lowest level, the **ANS**, which deals with bodily states. A division can be drawn between the *central* ANS (**insula, amygdala, hypothalamus**, and several midbrain nuclei, including the **periaqueductal gray matter [PAG]**) and the *peripheral* ANS (the sympathetic nervous system, the parasympathetic nervous system, the neuroendocrine system, and the **enteric nervous system**, which controls digestion). We will first discuss the hypothalamus (literally, below the thalamus) because of its central role in mediation between the CNS and the body, and then discuss the midbrain nuclei. (The amygdala and insula are at higher levels in the model and are discussed later.) The hypothalamus has two-way connections to virtually all of the rest of the CNS, and to every organ in the body, allowing it to act as an integrative center that controls the pANS to maintain homeostasis (Card et al., 2008). The hypothalamus controls the so-called "fight-or-flight" response by activating the sympathetic portion of the pANS, which acts on multiple body organs to prepare the organism for an emergency defensive response (by increasing heart rate, dilating the pupils of the eyes, inhibiting salivation and digestion, and promoting elimination of bodily wastes). Importantly, in normal function, the hypothalamus returns the pANS to the ordinary baseline or resting state by activating the parasympathetic portion of the pANS, which has an opposite effect on these body organs. The hypothalamus also controls the neuroendocrine system, which regulates numerous basic bodily states including hunger, thirst, stress, sex, sleep, thermoregulation, and aspects of immune function. The hypothalamus lies beneath the thalamus and above the optic chiasm and consists of many distinct nuclei. These nuclei regulate different bodily functions by secreting both peptides (such as oxytocin and vasopressin) and so-called "releasing hormones" into the portal connecting the hypothalamus to the pituitary. These peptides and releasing hormones cause the pituitary to release other hormones into the bloodstream so they can reach peripheral organs. Examples of releasing hormones include gonadotropin-releasing hormome (GnRH), involved in sexual differentiation; corticotropin-releasing hormone (CRH), involved in the stress response; and growth-hormone-releasing hormone (GHRH).

The midbrain nuclei in the ANS include the PAG and four nuclei that modulate forebrain activity by releasing neurotransmitters that are familiar targets of psychiatric medications: (1) the **locus coeruleus (LC)**, the source of norepinephrine projections; (2) **raphe nuclei (RN)**, the source of serotoninergic projections; (3) the **substantia nigra (SN)**, which is the source of the dopaminergic projection to the dorsal striatum (and which degenerates in PD); and (4) the **ventral tegmental area (VTA)**, the source of dopaminergic projections to the ventral striatum (nucleus accumbens [NAcc]), olfactory bulb, amygdala, hippocampus, anterior cingulate gyrus (ACG), and all three divisions of the PFC: lateral, medial, and orbital. Hence, these four nuclei can modulate the motivational state of the entire forebrain. Because each receives descending projections from the PFC, motivational state can be adjusted to match current action plans. The name of the PAG derives from the fact that it is a band of gray matter around the cerebral aqueduct in the midbrain. The PAG, like the hypothalamus, is involved in several basic motivational states and related behaviors including pain and analgesia, fear, lordosis (female posture for sex), basic vocalizations, and cardiovascular functioning. The PAG projects to the VTA, and possibly the three other nuclei discussed here (SN, LC, and RN). Panksepp (1998) has identified seven different midbrain mammalian circuits in the PAG and related structures involved in the core affective processes of seeking, rage, fear, panic, lust, care, and play. Panksepp's work and that of other affective neuroscientists support an evolutionary origin for core human emotions, so his theory is a discrete emotion theory, as is Ekman's (Ekman, 2003) and Izard's (1992). A competing social construction theory of emotions (Barrett, 2012) argues against innate discrete emotions because the predicted one-to-one correspondences between brain sites and emotional experiences do not hold up empirically and because emotional experiences and expressions are always affected by socialization (each emotion is socially real but is not distinct without socialization). It is not clear whether this argument also applies to homeostatic affects like physical pain or taste aversion, which are present in neonates and across species. In the hierarchical model presented here, midbrain circuits interact with other levels of the state regulation system, and with socialization, to determine experience and behavior. So, it may be that whether a motivational state is discrete or not depends on which level in this hierarchy is being examined.

At the next level in the model are two structures, the **amygdala** and **nucleus accumbens (NAcc)**, that represent the implicit hedonic tone of states and can guide behavior without conscious awareness. The amygdala (named with the Latin word for "almond" because of its shape) is a small structure located anterior to the hippocampus in the medial temporal lobe (MTL). It consists of four nuclei that can be divided into two functional groups: a basolateral amygdala complex (consisting of three nuclei: lateral, basolateral, and basomedial) and the central nucleus of the amygdala. The basolateral complex is, broadly speaking, the input portion of the amygdala and has reciprocal connections with sensory thalamus, hippocampus, and neocortex, as well as the NAcc, discussed next. The connections with the hippocampus allow the emotional significance of an episode to influence the strength of memory consolidation. The central nucleus is the output portion of the amygdala and exerts top-down control over the ANS through connections to the hypothalamus, the PAG, and other structures. This anatomy permits the amygdala to process emotionally relevant sensory inputs and coordinate an appropriate behavioral and autonomic response.

In fMRI studies of typical adults, the amygdala is activated by facial expression of the negative emotions of anger and fear. Moreover, this activation can be elicited subliminally (Whalen et al., 1998). The most studied function of the amygdala in state regulation is fear conditioning (LaBar & LeDoux, 2003), through which anticipatory bodily responses can be elicited by a previously neutral stimulus after as little as one pairing (hence called "one-trial learning"). Lesion studies in humans and other animals have confirmed that the amygdala is necessary for fear conditioning. For instance, a human patient with a discrete amygdala lesion was found to be incapable of fear conditioning, even though he formed an episodic memory for the fear conditioning procedure. In contrast, a patient with a discrete hippocampal lesion had normal fear conditioning, despite lacking any memory of the conditioning procedure (Bechara et al., 1995). Typical humans can acquire a conditioned fear through verbal instruction alone (e.g., the blue square might lead to a shock), and the amygdala is activated in instructed fear conditioning (Phelps et al., 2001).

The amygdala is not exclusively concerned with the emotion of fear; it also has a role in reward-based learning through its connections with NA (Stuber, Britt, & Bonci, 2011). The amygdala responds to positive stimuli, as well as intense stimuli (e.g., odors) regardless of valence, although there are conflicting results regarding whether valence or emotional intensity is more important in activating the amygdala (Banich & Compton, 2011).

The other structure at this implicit level of the model is the NAcc, which is more strongly involved in positive motivational states than the amygdala. The Latin word *accumbens* means "leaning" and the NAcc was so named because it appears to be leaning against the septum. The NAcc and the olfactory tubercle compose the ventral striatum, because they are the lower or ventral part of the striatum. The NAcc has connections to other structures involved in state regulation, which are also interconnected. It receives dopaminergic projections from the VTA, top-down inputs from the PFC, inputs from CA1 cells in the hippocampus, and, importantly for the model presented here, inputs from the amygdala. Its connection with the hippocampus allows it to play a role in memory consolidation similar to that played by the amygdala. Its role in reward processing was discovered by Olds and Milner (1954) in a brain stimulation study of rats. The rats could stimulate the median forebrain bundle, of which the NAcc is an important part, by pressing a lever connected to an implanted electrode and would continue pressing the lever as long as they could because it was presumably pleasurable. Hence, the median forebrain bundle and eventually the NA became known as the "pleasure center" of the brain, although later research has refined our understanding of the role of the NAcc in reward processing, and we now understand that continual lever pressing by the rats was because their "seeking" or "wanting" circuit was activated, not their pleasure center. The NAcc is divided into a core and shell portion, with the core associated with implicit wanting or seeking and the shell associated with implicit liking (Berridge, 2003). This distinction between implicit wanting and liking, originally discovered by Panksepp (Panksepp & Biven, 2012), is psychologically important, because we can seek things we do not like (as in nicotine and other addictions) and we can like things but still not seek them (as in a disorder like schizophrenia, where patients have a liking response to a rewarding taste, such as chocolate, but do not seek chocolate because of their avolition/abulia). Neuroimaging studies in humans have demonstrated that the NAcc is activated by various rewarding stimuli, including sweet juice, money, attractive faces, pleasant pictures and music, and addictive substances in people who are addicted to them (Banich & Compton, 2011; Sabatinelli, Bradley, Lang, Costa, & Versace, 2007), but the resolution of fMRI does not allow us to determine whether this is because of wanting, liking, or both. Positive mental imagery also activates the NAcc (Costa, Lang, Sabatinelli, Versace, & Bradley, 2010). The NAcc is also a key structure involved in the placebo effect.

We have already covered the key structure at the next level of the hierarchical model in Table 11.1, the dorsal striatum, which is involved in learning to approach or avoid various stimuli. At the next level, we come to the insula (the Latin word for "island"), which plays a key role in interoception, the perception of internal motivational states. The insula is a part of the neocortex that is folded beneath the sylvian fissure on each side of the brain, making it an "island" of neocortex underneath the neocortical surface. The insula receives interoceptive inputs from the thalamus, allowing it to represent these internal states consciously, and has outputs to other structures in Table 11.1, including the amygdala, the ventral striatum, and the orbitofrontal cortex (OFC). Interoceptive states that produce insula activation include (1) bodily states like heartbeat and gastric and bladder distension (related to the motivational state of elimination); (2) the negatively valenced states of pain (both physical and psychological) and the social emotion of disgust; and (3) the positively valenced states of craving rewards, like food and addictive substances. Not surprisingly, the insula is implicated in both addiction to drugs and eating disorders.

The two remaining structures to discuss in Table 11.1 are the subgenual cingulate gyrus (SGCG; Brodmann's area 25), and the ventromedial

PFC (vmPFC). The ventral PFC, DLPFC, and ACG have already been discussed in Chapter 10. The SGCG is part of the cingulate (from the Latin word for "girdle") gyrus, which wraps around the corpus callosum from front to rear. The genual portion of the corpus callosum is its anterior curve adjacent to medial PFC, and the portion of the cingulate gyrus beneath it is called subgenual, placing it in close proximity to some of the other motivational structures discussed here. It has a high concentration of serotonin receptors and is connected to other motivational structures, including the midbrain nuclei, the hypothalamus, the amygdala, and insula, all discussed earlier, and to the hippocampus. Mayberg (1997) published an influential paper identifying SGCG as a "gateway" structure in mood regulation, positing that major depression was due to an imbalance between overactivity in the SGCG and insufficient top-down control by the DLPFC and ACG. As will be discussed later, she tested this theory by using deep brain stimulation of the SGCG to relieve intractable depression (Mayberg et al., 2005).

The vmPFC is part of the much larger Brodmann's area 10 and some authors include medial orbital frontal cortex in their definition of vmPFC. Damasio and colleagues documented that damage to the vmPFC produces deficits in affective decision making, as discussed in Chapter 10. More recently, Wager and colleagues (e.g., Roy, Shohamy, & Wager, 2012) have shown that the vmPFC is activated in numerous tasks involving self-representations, including affective decision-making tasks. They hypothesize that this part of the brain is not necessary for affective responses, unlike many of the other structures discussed here, but is critical for regulating affective responses with conceptual information about self-relevant outcomes.

Now I will describe in more detail what the model in Table 11.1 says about how the brain accomplishes state regulation. First, we can draw a rough boundary line between the top three and bottom three levels of the model with respect to consciousness. The top three structures are involved in the conscious experience of motivational states and in their conscious regulation. The bottom three levels can operate automatically or implicitly. A key principle in the model is competition between states with positive and negative valences, and it is assumed that oppositely valenced states are usually mutually exclusive. More generally, various goals of the organism and the states associated with them are often in conflict, and this competition is resolved by interactions among all levels of the system, so that the organism arrives at a state and relevant action that is optimal for the current context. As discussed in Chapter 10, a key principle of

TABLE 11.1. Hierarchical Model of State Regulation

	Conceptual model	Neural structures
	Cognitive control (cold EF)	DLPFC and ACG
	Affective appraisal and regulation (hot EF)	vmPFC and SGCG
	Interoception	Insula
	Implicit approach–avoidance learning	Dorsal striatum
	Implicit hedonic tone (e.g., liking vs. disliking)	NAcc and amygdala
	Bodily states	Hypothalamus, PAG, and pANS

(Arrow labeled "Consciousness" pointing upward along the left side of the table.)

action selection is its relentless seriality; that is, we generally can only do one thing at a time. As we will see later, a problem in state regulation can arise at any level in the model, from the peripheral endocrine system all the way up to the level of cognitive control, and interactions to resolve these problems can be at all levels as well.

To understand disorders of state regulation, we need to understand why the system sometimes fails to return to homeostasis. One reason is that intense affective experiences, both positive and negative, can lead to pathological emotional responding, making it much easier for the system to return to that intense state instead of returning to homeostasis. We will discuss disorders of state regulation in more detail later in this chapter.

TYPICAL DEVELOPMENT

The development of state regulation is one of the primary tasks in infancy and early childhood, and crucially depends on interactions with parents and other caregivers. Attachment is fundamental to state regulation and emotional development. As any parent can attest, the first few months of a child's life are largely spent trying to establish regular routines of sleeping and feeding, and soothing a crying or overexcited baby. Sander (1964) studied how these routines get established in typical development and described the first 3 months of life as the phase of physiological regulation. As described in Berk (2005), newborns have two basic global arousal states, approach and withdrawal, and the perception and production of discrete emotions as social signals has not yet developed.

Nonetheless, neonates have a very important, innate, foundational social skill. They can imitate tongue protrusion and a few other gestures made by adults (Meltzoff & Moore, 1977). The later discovery of "mirror neurons" in Broca's area and other parts of the human and monkey brain have provided a neural mechanism for imitation. Mirror neurons are active both when a person is observing an action performed by another and when that person is performing the same action. To support neonatal imitation, some mirror neurons in the brain must be functional at birth, allowing the child to accomplish the difficult computational task of mapping seen movements made by another onto motor commands for the infant's own body. This very basic self–other correspondence is the foundation for solving the "other minds problem" and for developing self–other correspondences first in emotions and bodily states, then in attention, intention, and finally belief. So, social cognition has an innate foundation but then develops through interactions with others.

As discussed earlier, in Chapter 6, newborns also appear to have an innate preference for face-like stimuli, and then develop facial recognition skills over the coming months and years. These face-like stimuli have two "eyes." More recent research has found that neonates prefer a face with a direct gaze over a face with an averted gaze, and that direct gaze has a distinct neuroimaging signature in neonates (see review in Johnson & de Haan, 2011). In adults, an important structure in gaze processing is the superior temporal sulcus (STS), which is part of the social brain (for a review, see Adolphs, 2003).

Around 2 to 3 months of age, infants develop a social smile and use it to make bids for adults' attention. They also begin to make more eye-to-eye contact, mimic facial and vocal expressions of adults, and embark on the phase of reciprocal social–affective exchange in Sander's (1964) account. Part of the prelanguage "dialogue" between parents and infants consists of exchanges of what Stern (1985) calls "vitality affects." Vitality affects are different from discrete emotions like joy and fear, and refer to the activation contours of motions and voices that can relate to changes in internal states. Parents interact with lots of "oohs and ahs," exaggerated facial and manual gestures, and exaggerated prosody (called "motherese") when talking to infants. Preverbal babies can coo and make rising or falling sounds to match or improvise upon the parent's vocal and manual gestures, and then the parent can answer back. These young infants and their parents are having protoconversations, where the topic of conversation is usually about bodily states. These affective exchanges are the beginning of intersubjectivity, the insight that other humans have internal subjective states similar to one's own. So, in Stern's (1985) account, the infant begins to "solve" the other minds problem through imitative and affective exchanges.

In the second half of the first year of life, infants begin to become aware of a more cognitive state that can be shared with another person, the state of attention. Infants develop what is called "joint attention," that is, sharing attention to an external object of interest with another person. Infants learn to follow an adult's gaze or pointing gesture toward an external object and to initiate a gaze or a point and then check back to see if the adult is gazing there. In a joint attention exchange, an infant "secures reference" with a partner through what are called **protodeclarative gestures**, the nonverbal equivalent of "Look, Mom, there's a dog!" Protodeclarative gestures are distinct from **protoimperative gestures**, the use of voice and hand gestures to request or demand a desired object, such as food or a toy.

The development of language in the second year of life builds on joint attention and allows the toddler to have a much more diverse and less ambiguous method of securing reference with a communicative partner. During the second year, toddlers also develop an understanding of their own and others' intentions. Once discovered, their will must be practiced, sometimes to the distress of their parents when faced with the tantrums that mark the "terrible 2's."

The final preschool milestone in the development of intersubjectivity is the understanding of false belief, which develops around age 4. Preschoolers come to understand that their own and others' beliefs can be mistaken and that individuals can have different beliefs. This mentalizing activity has been studied with fMRI in both adults and children, and one consensus brain area activated by theory of mind tasks is the medial PFC (mPFC; see Banich & Compton, 2011, and Johnson & de Haan, 2011, for reviews). However, children differ from adults in consistently showing greater mPFC activity and less activity in posterior portions of the social brain, such as the STS. This developmental shift from mPFC to posterior cortex is partly consistent with the interactive specialization view of brain development, in which the PFC is more involved when learning a new skill, which once learned is mediated by posterior cortex. However, the persisting mPFC activity in adults on mentalizing tasks indicates that this skill cannot be completely automated or delegated to posterior cortex. Simulation of another's mental states may always require reference to one's own mental states, which, as described earlier, are represented in vmPFC. Even though preschoolers have some grasp of theory of mind (or "first-order theory of mind," as indexed by standard false belief tasks), the understanding of theory of mind continues to develop at least into young adulthood, if not beyond. Tasks have been developed that tap secondary theory of mind, in which one actor thinks about what a second actor thinks. Because of recursion, one can imagine third- and higher-order theory of mind problems that go well beyond most adults' abilities to understand, but can be involved in high-level diplomacy and espionage (Germany thinks that Greece thinks that Germany thinks, etc., etc.). Mentalizing also obviously develops in other ways besides understanding false belief.

Much of the foregoing is relevant for understanding autism, which is a neurodevelopmental disorder in which there are impairments in many but not all of the social–emotional milestones just discussed. Children with autism are impaired in imitation, joint attention, language, theory of mind, and some aspects of processing and regulating emotions. In contrast, they do not appear to be impaired in the development of the social smile. A more extensive review of autism is contained in Pennington (2009); in other parts of this book we discuss autism as an example of a disorder in which there is abnormal brain connectivity. But much remains to be learned about how alterations in brain development lead to the behaviors that characterize autism. I think autism is the least well-explained disorder in this book.

DISORDERS

To explain disorders of state regulation, we will use the model presented in Table 11.1. These disorders are due to imbalance, either *vertical* or *horizontal*. Vertical imbalance is an imbalance between top-down control and bottom-up activation, and vertical imbalances can occur between any two levels in the model. Vertical imbalance has been the main model to explain many psychopathologies, sometimes tautologically (e.g., "disorder X represents a failure of inhibition or impulse control"). Just saying that a given act or person is impulsive or disinhibited is only a description; to be explanatory, we must be able to say why the individual failed to inhibit an inappropriate action. To do this, we need to be able to measure the strength of *both* top-down regulation and bottom-up activation, which can be very difficult to do. In many neuroimaging studies of disorders like depression or anxiety, top-down regulation is operationalized as activity in the PFC, and bottom-up activation is operationalized as activity in sub-cortical structures that mediate motivational states, such as the amygdala. Such studies often find reduced PFC activation and increased activity in a relevant subcortical structure, such as the amygdala in anxiety and depression. But such studies do not tell us how the vertical imbalance arose. Did it start with too much bottom-up activation, or too little top-down regulation, or some combination of the two?

Horizontal imbalance is an imbalance between valences at the same level. Horizontal imbalance is used less frequently as an explanation for psychopathologies, but is highly relevant for understanding mood, anxiety, and addictive disorders. As we saw in Chapter 10, horizontal imbalance between the striatal go and no-go pathways provided a good explanation for the symptoms of PD and TS. To explain disorders of state regulation, we need to add other structures to the cortical–striatal loop model, as explained earlier in discussing the model in Table 11.1. The key extra structures are those at the bottom two levels of the model, bodily states (hypothalamus, midbrain gray nuclei and PAG, and pANS) and implicit hedonic tone (amygdala and NAcc), as well as at the level of interoception (insula) and affective appraisal and regulation (vmPFC and SGCG).

A disorder can arise due to imbalance at any level of the system, from the cognitive to the pANS, but once there is an imbalance at any level, it propagates to all the other levels. Just as typical motivational states organize the whole system to prepare for an appropriate action, an imbalance in motivational state captures the whole system, which then cannot return to homeostasis. So a key prediction of this model is that any disorder of state regulation should have a characteristic signature at every level in Table 11.1.

As mentioned earlier, learning or plasticity occurs throughout the system, but some learning represents pathological plasticity (similar to kindling). The more the system is in an extreme state, the easier it is to return to that state and everything associated with it (perceptual cues, habits, and memories). Often the person becomes fixated on the abnormal state (e.g., a fear, a craving, or a mood), ruminates about it to try to regulate it, but paradoxically becomes trapped in repetitive thoughts and actions to attempt to alleviate that state.

As discussed earlier, Ohman (2000) proposed that the evolutionary advantage of rapid emotional conditioning, especially fear conditioning, has left us with a vulnerability to anxiety disorders. As summarized in

Pennington (2002), in this theory, the anxiety response is an evolved, automatic, defensive response meant to deal with threats to survival (i.e., the classic fight-or-flight response). In the realistically threatening environment in which humans evolved, there was much more selection pressure against false negatives in the activation of this response (e.g., failing to run from a tiger) than against false positives (e.g., running from one's own shadow). Consequently, part of our evolutionary heritage is an easily triggered anxiety response. This evolutionary perspective may help explain why anxiety disorders are the most common of all psychopathologies.

Another requirement for such a response is that it should detect potential threats quickly. Considerable empirical work by Ohman and others (reviewed in Ohman, 2000), using backward masking and divided attention paradigms, demonstrates rapid, nonconscious processing of threat stimuli, which is more pronounced in individuals with anxiety disorders. The preattentive, nonconscious processing of threat stimuli is consistent with LeDoux's model (LaBar & LeDoux, 1996) of amygdala functioning, in which certain threat stimuli can reach the amygdala without first being processed by the cortex.

Hence, evolution has prepared us to be more anxious than we need to be, especially given the relative safety of modern life, and to rapidly and unconsciously process signs of threat. Genetically influenced individual differences in this evolved anxiety response mean that some people will be particularly prone to having the anxiety response triggered by the wrong context, as in phobias, or with too low a threshold, as in panic disorder (Ohman, 2000). Once such a false-positive anxiety response occurs, the quickness of fear conditioning, the misattribution of the sufferer (e.g., "I'm going to die"), and the avoidance of subsequent exposure all make a recurrence more likely.

A similar argument can be made for depression, namely that it often begins with an intense stress response (such as a significant loss). As summarized in Pennington (2002), genetic studies provide a basis for understanding individual differences in susceptibility to depression. Stress and loss can cause depression, and early stress and loss can create a lasting vulnerability, as well as exacerbating vulnerability in individuals at genetic risk. Affect regulation is a key early developmental task, as well as a lifelong one, and depends crucially on socialization. Self-cognitions and attributional style also make important contributions to affect regulation, as do social support, exercise, sleep, nutrition, and certain illnesses. Perhaps because of the evolutionary advantage provided by being able to quickly mobilize a stress response, the amygdala and the hypothalamus–pituitary–adrenocortical (HPA) axis have a built-in Achilles' heel: they are easily overactivated. The immune system provides an interesting parallel; disorders involving an exaggerated immune response (e.g., allergies) are quite common. Natural selection quickly weeds out genes for weak immune responses or slow fear conditioning, but there is probably little selection pressure against extremes in the opposite direction.

What we understand less well about the two mood disorders major depressive disorder (MDD) and bipolar disorder (BPD) is their episodic course. That is, we do not know why the system gets "stuck" in an abnormal mood state, and especially why that mood state can spontaneously remit. We do understand much better what risk factors trigger episodes in MDD and BPD. For instance, life events characterized by stress and loss trigger episodes of MDD, whereas life events of high goal attainment or goal frustration trigger episodes of BPD (Urosevic, Abramson, Harmon-Jones, & Alloy, 2008). The kindling theory provides an explanation for why subsequent episodes require less of a trigger than earlier ones. But how does the system spontaneously get unstuck? All we can say is that the nervous system in a person with a mood disorder still strives for homeostasis, and thus some eventually get "unstuck" from an extreme mood state, but we know virtually nothing about the mechanisms of spontaneous remission.

Disorders of state regulation vary along three dimensions: valence (positive or negative), time course (acute, episodic, or chronic), and specificity of the trigger (Table 11.2). If we leave out time course, we can have an even simpler model (see Figure 11.1 on p. 192). These models are based on Gray's (1982) behavioral activation and inhibition systems (BAS and BIS) model of anxiety, and its extension to MD and BPD (Depue & Iacono, 1989; Urosevic et al., 2008). The BAS is associated with positive affect and approach behavior and the BIS with negative affect, especially fear, and avoidance behavior. In Gray's BAS/BIS model, anxiety and mood disorders are explained by a pattern of overactivity or underactivity in each system. Interestingly, questionnaire measures of BAS and BIS activity predicted later BPD and MDD episodes, respectively, in a longitudinal study of patients with histories of those two disorders (Alloy et al., 2008).

It is important to note that although the two valences are ordinarily mutually inhibitory, they are not mutually exclusive because they are handled by different systems. For instance, in BPD there can be mixed states (mania with high anxiety), with overactivity of both the BAS and BIS. We will now discuss available research on the disorders in Table 11.2 at each of the six levels in Table 11.1.

TABLE 11.2. Disorders of State Regulation

	Behavioral activation system	Behavioral inhibition system	Time course	Specificity
Mania	Overactivated	Normal/ overactivated	Episodic	General
Depression	Extremely underactivated	Overactivated	Episodic	General
Specific phobias	Normal except with trigger	Overactivated	Acute	Specific
Panic	Normal except with trigger	Extremely overactivated	Acute	Specific
Posttraumatic stress disorder	Normal except with trigger	Overactivated	Acute	Specific
Agoraphobia	Underactivated	Overactivated	More chronic	Less specific
Generalized anxiety disorder	Underactivated	Overactivated	More chronic	Less specific
Addiction	Overactivated	Underactivated	Chronic	Specific

Bodily States

Each of these disorders has autonomic symptoms whose duration is related to the chronicity and specificity of the disorder. In simple phobias, there is temporary sympathetic nervous system overactivity in the presence of the feared object or when thinking about it. In a chronic, general disorder like major depression (MDD), there are persisting and pervasive autonomic disturbances in sleep, appetite, and sexual desire, as well as a well-documented exaggerated stress response in the HPA axis (Nemeroff, 1998). In a manic episode, most of these autonomic symptoms have an opposite profile to that observed in MDD. There is a markedly reduced need for sleep and an increase in appetite and sexual desire.

Changes in the autonomic system can be a primary etiology of MDD, as seen in Cushing syndrome, thyroiditis (which results in low thyroid hormone), and postpartum depression (in which decreases in estrogen, progesterone, and thyroid hormone are thought to play a role). Hyperthyroidism (too much thyroid hormone) produces symptoms of anxiety.

Implicit Hedonic Tone

Increased amygdala activity, especially in response to sad or fearful faces, in fMRI studies is a well-replicated finding in MDD (Banich & Compton, 2011; Drevets, Price, & Furey, 2008) and anxiety disorders (Banich & Compton, 2011; Etkin & Wager, 2010). In contrast, reduced NAcc activity is found in several fMRI studies of MDD (Banich & Compton, 2011), and this reduction is correlated with the degree of anhedonia. Although fMRI studies of anxiety disorders do not seem to focus on NAcc activity, the model presented in Table 11.1 implies that NAcc activity should be normal in specific phobias, panic disorder, and PTSD, and somewhat decreased in agoraphobia and generalized anxiety disorder (GAD), though less decreased than in MDD. In contrast, the model predicts that NAcc activity should be increased in mania. There are few studies of this topic, but a recent fMRI study of euthymic (remitted) patients with bipolar I disorder (Nusslock et al., 2012) found increased activity in these patients, compared to controls, in the ventral striatum and OFC during anticipation (but not receipt) of reward in a card guessing task. Incidentally, both the liking and wanting associated with the NAcc and dorsal striatum are involved in the brain's processing of food rewards and may play a role in eating disorders (Berridge, 2009).

Implicit Approach–Avoidance Learning

This system has been less explored in these disorders, although there is some research on go versus no-go learning in addiction (Maia & Frank, 2011) and a discussion of how such implicit learning might explain learned helplessness in MDD (Montague, Dolan, Friston, & Dayan, 2012). Chase et al. (2010) found null behavioral results in patients with MDD on the probabilistic learning task used in Frank et al. (2004) with patients with PD. In a follow-up study of MDD by this same group, Cavanagh, Bismark, Frank, and Allen (2011) recorded error-related negativity (ERN) with an EEG study and found a higher-amplitude ERN signal in the MDD group compared to controls and a stronger relation between ERN and avoidance learning.

Interoception

Hamilton, Chen, Thomason, Schwartz, and Gotlib (2012) conducted a recent meta-analysis of neuroimaging studies of response to negative stimuli by patients with MDD. They found overactivity in several parts

	Approach	Avoid
Low Generalization	Specific Addictions	Specific Phobia
High Generalization	Bipolar Disorder	Major Depressive Disorder

FIGURE 11.1. State regulation disorders. Common state regulation disorders vary on approach–avoidance and generalization dimensions. For example, avoidance predominates in depression and generalizes across most situations.

of the motivation system including in the pulvinar nucleus of the thalamus (which projects to the amygdala), the amygdala itself, the insula, and the ACG. C. L. McGrath et al. (2013) found that anterior insula activation as measured by PET scan, predicted which treatment for MDD (cognitive-behavioral therapy [CBT] versus medication with escitalopram (Lexapro), a commonly used SSRI in the treatment of MDD) resulted in treatment success (remission). In this RCT of the two treatments (CBT versus medication), PET was used prior to treatment to measure regional blood flow to candidate regions of the brain, including the anterior insula. After treatment, patients were divided into four groups based on which treatment they received (CBT vs. medication) and treatment response (remitted vs. not remitted). These researchers found a crossover interaction effect, such that anterior insula hypermetabolism (increased blood flow relative to whole brain blood flow) predicted treatment success with medication, whereas anterior insula hypometabolism (decreased relative blood flow) predicted treatment success with CBT. One can speculate that patients with an overactive insula are self-monitoring too much (i.e., ruminating) and hence benefit from a medication known to reduce rumination. In contrast, patients with an underactive insula are self-monitoring too little and hence benefit from a treatment known to promote healthy self-monitoring. This study provides further evidence for the role of the insula in MDD, and if replicated, could help in selecting the most appropriate treatment for patients with MDD. Future research should also measure brain metabolism before and after treatment to test whether the expected changes in insula activity accompanied remission.

Insula overactivity to negative stimuli has also been found in anxiety disorders. Based on these findings, Paulus and Stein (2006) have proposed a model of anxiety proneness in which an exaggerated interoceptive prediction signal of possible future negative events leads to rumination.

Naqvi and Bechara (2009) reviewed evidence bearing on the role of the insula in addiction, in which the BAS is overactive. This evidence includes 16 functional imaging studies of conscious, cue-induced drug urges in addicts. Increased insula activation relative to baseline was present in all studies, whereas altered activation in structures that mediate implicit hedonic tone (amygdala and NAcc) was only found in about a third of the studies. This pattern of results supports the role of the insula in conscious urges for addictive substances. (In about two-thirds of the studies, there was altered activity in three structures involved in the regulation of addictive behaviors: DLPFC, OFC, and ACG). Naqvi and Bechara (2009) also reported dramatic cessations of addiction after insula lesions in humans and suppression of addiction by anesthesia in rats. Based on these empirical results, they proposed a model of addiction in which interoceptive predictive signals in the insula associated with substance use (the rituals and sensory experiences, not just the dopamine reward itself) promote the maintenance of addictive behaviors.

Affective Appraisal and Regulation

The main result at this level of the model is increased activity of SGCG in MDD (Drevets et al., 2008; Mayberg, 1997). As mentioned earlier, deep brain stimulation of inhibitory pathways regulating this structure can reduce its activity and effectively treat intractable MDD (Mayberg et al., 2005). Unlike null results for specific phobia and social anxiety, the meta-analysis by Etkin and Wager (2007) found underactivation of vmPFC in PTSD, consistent with a failure to use representations of the self (which are mediated by vmPFC) to regulate anxiety.

Cognitive Control

Decreased structural volumes and functional activity in DLPFC are well-documented correlates of MDD (see reviews in Banich & Compton, 2011; Drevets et al., 2008) and consistent with decreased top-down regulation posited by a vertical imbalance model of MDD (Gotlib & Hamilton, 2008). The other side of this vertical imbalance is the well-documented overactivity in bottom-up activation of the amygdala and other BIS structures, as reviewed earlier. Similar DLPFC reductions are also found in BPD (Drevets et al., 2008). In contrast, decreased activity in these cognitive control structures is not a consistent finding in anxiety disorders

(Etkin & Wager, 2007), except for consistent underactivation of ACG in PTSD. Studies of other anxiety disorders sometimes find increases in ACG activity, consistent with oversensitivity to threat and errors (Banich & Compton, 2011). Increased ACG activity in response to negative stimuli is a consistent finding in MDD in the meta-analysis performed by Hamilton et al. (2012).

CHAPTER SUMMARY

In general, functional neuroimaging and other results reviewed here are consistent with the model of state regulation disorders presented in Tables 11.1 and 11.2, and document both vertical and horizontal imbalance in these disorders. With few exceptions, the results reviewed here are correlational rather than experimental, so they do not address the question discussed earlier of which changes in this hierarchical model of state regulation are causal in the various disorders considered here.

EXERCISES

1. Go to *http://old.neurosynth.org/terms* and enter the term "happy." Adjust the scroll bars on the right sides of the three slice perspectives to find areas of activation. What brain structures are implicated, and at which level do they fall in the model in Table 11.1? What do you find if you type in "sad" or "fear"?

2. Agoraphobia is the fear of crowded spaces or enclosed public places. Thus, it closely resembles a specific phobia. However, there are important differences between agoraphobia and specific phobia in the model in Table 11.2. Using what you've learned from the Table 11.1 model and the discussion on learning, plasticity, and kindling, discuss how these differences arise.

CHAPTER 12

■■■■■■■

Global Disorders

DEFINITION

In this last chapter of Part II, we will consider disorders that affect multiple domains of the functions described in the previous chapters. These disorders are global (or general) because they typically produce a large deficit in both adaptive functioning and in overall IQ. However, their group profiles vary across different specific domains of neuropsychological functions. So, these global disorders shed light on the different ways in which IQ and adaptive behavior can be disrupted.

BRAIN MECHANISMS

Intelligence and adaptive behavior require the integrated functions of many parts of the brain. Neuroimaging studies have identified an important role for the PFC (and the parietal cortex in fluid intelligence, or novel problem solving), but functional and structural connectivity are also important. All the global disorders considered here impair executive functions mediated by the PFC, and they more variably impair other cognitive functions, such as language and aspects of memory.

TYPICAL DEVELOPMENT

Both intelligence and adaptive behavior have a protracted developmental course, with some aspects (e.g., fluid intelligence) reaching a lifetime peak in young adulthood, and others (e.g., social judgment and acquired knowledge, which is called "crystallized intelligence") continuing to develop well into maturity. Both functional and structural connectivity, as well as gray matter pruning, continue to develop at least into young adulthood and are related to both developmental and individual differences in intelligence. In later life, a large proportion of adults are faced with the prospect of developing dementia before they die. Cognitive development and devolution in age affect some shared cognitive and brain processes. For instance, prefrontally mediated executive functions have a protracted development in childhood and adolescence and are the most vulnerable to both normal and pathological cognitive aging. Processing speed is similarly protracted in its development in youth and vulnerable in aging. Processing speed is mediated in part by white matter connectivity, which develops slowly in youth and declines with age.

DISORDERS

With one exception, the global disorders considered in this chapter fall into two broad categories based on age of onset: (1) intellectual disability (ID) syndromes, which are chronic neurodevelopmental disorders that are present from birth; and (2) dementia syndromes, which are neurodegenerative disorders whose onset is typically in adulthood, usually in old age. The one exception is acquired brain injury, which can occur across the lifespan and varies more widely in severity than ID or dementia syndromes. Repeated traumatic brain injuries (TBIs), usually from contact sports like boxing and football, may lead to a distinctive progressive dementia, called chronic traumatic encephalopathy (CTE), which is currently an active area of research.

Since nearly all of these global disorders have identified etiologies and/or neuropathology whose effects on their neuropsychology have been studied systematically, these disorders are often better understood than behaviorally defined disorders (like autism or schizophrenia) that also have a global effect on cognitive and adaptive functioning. Some of the global disorders in this chapter have provided fruitful analogies for understanding behaviorally defined disorders, and it is likely they will continue to do so. These global disorders also remind us that because of the interactivity of the brain, *every* disorder in this book is a mix of general and specific effects. What varies is the extent and severity of the general deficits.

ID Syndromes

We will begin with ID syndromes. Those mainly covered here are (1) Down syndrome (DS), (2) fragile X syndrome (FXS), and (3) Williams syndrome (WS), although I will briefly describe a few others. A more extensive review of these three syndromes can be found in Pennington (2009).

Down Syndrome

DS is the most prevalent (about 1 to 1.5 per 1000 live births) form of ID with a known genetic etiology (**nondisjunction** of chromosome 21). Because nondisjunction is not familial, the large majority (94%) of cases of DS are nonfamilial and the most well-documented risk factor for DS is greater maternal age. The genetic etiology of DS involves a whole extra chromosome (and an extra dose of the gene products of all its genes), so tracing the developmental pathways from genotype to phenotype is much more difficult in DS than in FXS or WS. Some progress is being made by developing mouse models of DS, which have varying degrees of trisomy for the mouse homologue of chromosome 21, and by applying what we already know about some of the genes on this chromosome. For instance, the gene for the amyloid precursor protein (APP) is on chromosome 21, and the extra dose of this gene is considered to be a significant risk factor for the high rate of early-onset Alzheimer's disease (AD) in DS. That is because amyloid plaques are part of the characteristic neuropathology of AD and are found in the brains of individuals with DS who have developed AD. Hence, DS is the clearest current example of how research on dementia and a neurodevelopmental ID can complement each other, although recent discoveries in FXS have pointed to a similar connection, as will be discussed below.

The extra dose of chromosome 21 genes in DS produces a characteristic physical, behavioral, and neurological phenotype, although it is important to remember that these phenotypes of DS are an *average* effect for groups with DS, and that there is a wide range of individual differences, as there are in other genetic and behavioral syndromes, as discussed earlier. For instance, some individuals with the DS genotype do not have ID because their IQ and adaptive behavior are better than the required cutoff for ID (at or below the second percentile).

Besides low IQ, the neuropsychological phenotype in DS includes performance below mental age level on verbal STM and language skills (such as syntax and articulation), verbal and visual spatial episodic LTM, and certain executive function (EF) tasks (e.g., Zelazo's dimensional card sorting task, which is a "junior" version of the Wisconsin Card Sorting Task, which elicits perseverative responding in patients with PFC lesions). Moreover, the *rate* of cognitive development is depressed in children with DS, resulting in a declining IQ.

The neurological phenotype in children and adults with DS includes **microcephaly** and differentially smaller volumes of the cerebellum, hippocampus, and PFC. These features all predate the later development of AD in DS, so the early and late neurological phenotypes likely have different genetic causes. Very little is known about actual brain development in DS because there are no longitudinal studies.

Although we can propose plausible brain–behavior relations between the neuroanatomical and neuropsychological phenotypes, such as the relationship of microcephaly to low IQ, decreased hippocampal volumes to episodic LTM deficits, and decreased PFC volume to EF deficits, these associations have not been systematically tested. So, we do not know which aspects of the neuroanatomical phenotype cause which aspects of the neuropsychological phenotype, and what the balance is between general and specific effects. Comparisons with other ID syndromes can address some of these questions. For instance, microcephaly alone cannot explain the verbal STM deficit in DS, because this deficit is not found in WS, even though both disorders share this brain phenotype.

Fragile X Syndrome

FXS is the most prevalent *inherited* form of ID, so unlike DS it is both genetic *and* familial. It has the simplest genetic etiology of these three syndromes, because it is a single-gene disorder, in which the FMR1 gene on the distal end of the long arm of the X chromosome becomes inactivated through **methylation**. Because FMR1 is on the X chromosome, FXS exhibits X-linked inheritance, in which males are more frequently and severely affected than females (because females have two X chromosomes, while males have only one). Although FXS is a single-gene disorder, its etiology is not as simple as that of a classic, Mendelian autosomal single-gene disorder like phenylketonuria (PKU). FXS has two important non-Mendelian features that have contributed to changes in our understanding of how genes work. It is an epigenetic disorder because it results from abnormal gene expression rather than a mutation in the coding portion (exons) of the FMR1 gene. This change in gene expression results from an accumulation across generations of repetitive, trinucleotide (CGG, in this case) repeats in noncoding portions of the FMR1 gene. Once the number of CGG repeats reaches a critical threshold of around 200, the whole FMR1 gene is methylated (by the attachment of CH3 molecules to the DNA), resulting in gene inactivation. Hence, FMRP, a gene product, critical for normal brain and physical development, is unavailable. FMRP is an RNA-binding protein that has a broad role in protein synthesis in the brain and affects dendritic spine maturation, synaptogenesis, and pruning of dendrites and synapses. These three processes are critical for early postnatal brain development, namely the process of experience-expectant synaptogenesis discussed earlier. The second non-Mendelian feature in the genetics of FXS is a parent-of-origin effect mediated by what is called **imprinting**, which also affects gene expression. In the case of FXS, the expansion of the number of CGG repeats is greater when the already expanded but subthreshold FMR1 gene is inherited from the mother rather than the father. Because of these non-Mendelian features, full FXS can appear abruptly in a family and appear to be a sporadic mutation.

FMRP binds to specific messenger RNAs [mRNAs], which transcribe the message in coding regions of genes in dendritic spines to down-regulate protein synthesis, so absence of FMRP leads to an excess of these proteins, thus affecting maturation of dendritic spines, and hence synaptogenesis and pruning. In particular, signaling by the metabotropic glutamate receptor (mGluR) is overactivated by the lack of FMRP, leading to an excess of the AMPA receptor (Garber, Visootsak, & Warren, 2008). Use of an mGluR antagonist has reversed some of the effects of FXS in tissue culture and animal models, so the prospect of a preventive treatment in humans is on the horizon. In sum, there has been considerable progress in understanding how the genetic mutation changes brain development in FXS and how some of these changes may be prevented.

In contrast to DS and WS, the neuroanatomical phenotype of FXS includes both smaller (cerebellar vermis) and larger (striatal–frontal) brain structures, the latter being consistent with reduced synaptic pruning. Recently, Hoeft et al. (2010) conducted a longitudinal neuroimaging study of boys with FXS from age 1 to age 3 to examine early brain development. Consistent with previous findings, they found a persistent reduction in the volume of the cerebellar vermis in contrast to a wider pattern of increased volumes in both gray and white matter. Specifically, they found a pattern of both early (caudate and fusiform gyri) and later (OFC and basal forebrain) gray matter increases, as well as greater white matter volumes that increased over the two time points in striatal–frontal areas. At a microscopic level, dendritic spines in FXS have been found to be immature and dense (Garber et al., 2008), consistent with the molecular mechanism described earlier.

The neuropsychological phenotype in FXS ID includes decline in IQ with age and prominent EF deficits, which in females with FXS are positively correlated to the degree of inactivation of the normal X chromosome. EF deficits are consistent with aspects of the neuroanatomical phenotype, such as the striatal–frontal differences, but this neuropsychological theory has not been systematically tested.

A new dementia syndrome resembling PD has been discovered in seemingly unaffected male FXS carriers once they get older (past age 50). This dementia is called FX tremor/ataxia syndrome. This discovery, similar to the link between DS and AD, demonstrates etiological connections between the two kinds of global disorders considered in this chapter: ID syndromes and dementias.

In sum, the discovery of the FMR1 gene about 20 years ago has led to dramatic progress in explaining FXS at several levels of analysis, spanning gene expression, brain development, neuropsychology, and behavior. FXS is thus the best-understood ID syndrome and arguably even the best-understood neurodevelopmental disorder, except for perhaps early treated PKU.

Williams Syndrome

This section draws on recent reviews of WS in Mervis and John (2010) and Pennington (2009). WS has a lower prevalence (1 per 7,500 live births) than DS or FXS, and like DS (and unlike FXS) is mostly nonfamilial. It is caused by a usually sporadic, contiguous microdeletion of the chromosomal region 7q11.23 on *one* of the two copies of chromosome 7 in the child's genotype (a deletion on *both* copies of the chromosome would be lethal for the fetus). So, WS, like DS, is due to an abnormal dose of normal gene products (deletion in WS and addition in DS) and not to an abnormal gene. This abnormal dose affects at least 25 genes, fewer than in DS (the critical DS region on chromosome 21 contains over 100 genes), but considerably more than FXS, in which only one gene product is absent (in affected males) or reduced (in affected females). One could reasonably ask why a segment consisting of these 25 or so genes is consistently deleted. The reason is that the deleted region is flanked by repetitive sequences, making it more susceptible to crossing-over errors in meiosis. Such errors result in either extra (nonviable), missing (i.e., deleted), or inverted copies of this region on one chromosome. Individuals with this inversion comprise about 7% of the population and are carriers who are five times more likely to transmit a deletion, and hence WS, to their children. Thus, in this minority of cases, WS is familial. Nonetheless, there are occasional partial deletions, so that some relatives of a WS proband can have partial versions of the syndrome, aiding in the task of relating specific genes in the deletion region to specific aspects of the WS phenotype. Nearly all genes in the deletion region have been identified and genotype–phenotype relations have been established for some of them. For instance, the ELN gene produces *elastin*, a protein important in connective tissue, and a reduced dose of this protein is involved in the cardiac and other connective tissue anomalies in WS. Other genes (LIMK1, CYLN2, GTF2I, and GTF2IRD1) are implicated in the cognitive phenotype of WS, discussed later.

A microaddition syndrome involving an extra dose of the same segment of chromosome 7q has recently been described; it is called 7q duplication syndrome (7q11.23dup). This syndrome is the genetic opposite of WS (a 50% dose of the products of the roughly 25 genes on 7q11.23 in WS versus a 150% dose in 7q11.23dup). Interestingly, the behavioral phenotypes of individuals with 7q11.23 dup syndrome, increased rates of autism, and severe speech dyspraxia is roughly the opposite of that found in WS, which is characterized by hypersociability and fluent speech (Sanders et al., 2011; Velleman & Mervis, 2011).

At the brain level, WS is characterized by overall microcephaly, as is DS, but the profile of affected structures differs from that found in DS. In WS, reductions are found in the parietal lobule, intraparietal sulcus, and occipital lobe, but not in the cerebellum (which has reduced volume in DS). Although hippocampal volume is not differentially reduced in WS (as it is in DS), the hippocampus exhibits a marked reduction in blood flow on functional neuroimaging scans. The other key functional neuroimaging findings document reduced dorsal stream activity in the parietal lobe and reduced amygdala activation in response to angry or fearful faces, but not to threatening or fearful scenes. These structural and functional neuroimaging findings can be related to two marked features of the neuropsychological phenotype in WS: (1) impairment in visuospatial processing (but not in face and object processing mediated by the ventral visual stream) and (2) social disinhibition, including an increased tendency to approach strangers.

In addition to a dramatic deficit in visuospatial processing (which is a relative strength in DS) and social disinhibition, other aspects of the neuropsychological phenotype in WS include the following:

1. A mean and stable IQ of about 60, which is in the lower portion of the mild ID range (55–70), in contrast to a declining and lower mean IQ in DS and FXS (where the mean IQ is in the moderate range of ID, at 40–55).
2. Overall language at mental age level and concrete vocabulary (e.g., as measured by the Peabody Picture Vocabulary Test) and verbal STM above mental age level, in contrast to DS.
3. Deficits in verbal and spatial LTM (Edgin, Pennington, & Mervis, 2010).
4. Deficits in verbal and spatial working memory (Edgin et al., 2010).

The LTM deficits are consistent with the hypoactivity of the hippocampus discussed earlier. The social and emotional phenotype is characterized by a paradoxical contrast between exaggerated sociability and empathy and exaggerated nonsocial anxiety, consistent with the amygdala findings discussed earlier. This phenotype is paradoxical because an anxious temperament usually results in reduced social approach.

In closing this section on WS, it is important to return to the issue of general versus specific deficits in ID syndromes. By definition (an IQ score < 70), ID syndromes have a general deficit in Spearman's g, so we should expect all cognitive skills to be depressed to a certain extent because all cognitive skills are correlated with g to some degree. As we have demonstrated, each ID syndrome considered here exhibits this global depression in cognitive skills, with some few specific skills being below or above mental age level, but none at cognitive age level. Hence, these contrasting cognitive profiles across ID syndromes provide evidence for some specificity to each syndrome that relates to its etiology, but not evidence for independent cognitive modules. For instance, it has been claimed that the double dissociation between Williams and Down syndromes with regard to language versus spatial functions provides support for an independent language module in the brain (Bellugi, Marks, Bihrle, & Sako, 1988). But neither "spared" skill in either syndrome is anywhere near an age-typical level of performance. So, as we have illustrated many times before, dissociations provide evidence for a degree of specialization in the cortex but not independent processes. The verbal and spatial LTM and working memory deficits found in WS in Edgin et al. (2010) were also found in the DS group. These results are important because they demonstrate that as the cognitive load (or one could say loading on g) for a cognitive task increases, the verbal versus spatial dissociation between DS and WS goes down. This result is contrary to the modular view of WS proposed by Bellugi et al. (1988). Also contrary to that view is the fact that overall language is at mental-age, not chronological-age, level in WS, and the contrasting language and spatial skills in WS are nonetheless correlated at about .50.

In summary, these three genetic IDs illustrate how we can provide a multilevel explanation of a behavioral disorder that links changes in the expression of particular genes to alterations in brain development, neuropsychology, and behavior. These three syndromes are part of the nearly 1,000 distinct genetic syndromes that cause ID. The multiplicity of possible genetic causes of ID is consistent with the highly polygenic etiology of normal variations in IQ, and the multiple brain regions that contribute to IQ. So, IDs are global developmental disorders that significantly lower IQ and adaptive function, which are general integrative functions of the CNS. In contrast, dementias are acquired neurological disorders in which these same integrative functions are lost later in life.

Dementia Syndromes

Alzheimer's Disease

Alzheimer's disease (AD) is the most prevalent degenerative dementia syndrome and accounts for about half of all cases of dementia. Nondegenerative dementias are less common overall and are due to an acquired brain insult and not to a progressive disease. The overall prevalence of AD in the United States is 1.9%, but prevalence rises dramatically after age 75. In U.S. adults ages 75–84, the prevalence is 19%; it rises to 42% in those 85 and older. AD is a cortical dementia, meaning that it selectively targets the cortex, with the hippocampus and related structures being most and earliest affected. As the disease progresses, secondary and tertiary areas of neocortex are more affected than primary areas, resulting in fewer simple neurological signs. AD is currently an incurable, fatal disease; the average survival time is about 7 years after the initial clinical diagnosis. However, the subclinical prodromal phase of the disease can begin decades before the clinical diagnosis. So, there has been considerable research on early detection of those at risk for later AD, using genetic, molecular, neurobehavioral, and neuroimaging measures.

The etiology of AD is multifactorial, with a heritability of about .60, meaning that there are also environmental risk factors for AD. As reviewed in Banich and Compton (2011), some of these environmental risk factors include smoking, cardiovascular disease, diabetes, and TBI.

Protective factors include use of nonsteroidal anti-inflammatory drugs (NSAIDs), education, exercise, estrogen replacement therapy in females, and mentally challenging work and leisure activities. Some of these protective factors are not necessarily exclusively environmental, since education and occupational status are moderately correlated with IQ, which is moderately heritable.

In terms of genetics, a small minority of cases (about 1/1000), marked by an earlier age of onset, have an autosomal dominant pattern of inheritance. At least three different genes can transmit AD in this Mendelian fashion: the amyloid precursor protein gene (APP), presenilin 1 (PSEN1), and presenilin 2 (PSEN2). Hence, there is genetic heterogeneity in dominantly transmitted AD, with each gene variant being largely sufficient to cause the disease, but none of them being necessary. The gene products of the latter two genes produce an enzyme that cleaves the APP protein. So, all three dominant genes for AD are involved in producing and processing amyloid. Since one hallmark of the neuropathology of AD is amyloid plaques in the brain, the connection of these genes to AD makes clear theoretical sense, although there is still considerable debate over whether changes in amyloid, tau (involved in the other key neuropathological feature of AD, neurofibrillary tangles), or neither are the primary cause of AD.

Since dominantly inherited cases are relatively rare, the bulk of the overall heritability of AD must be conveyed by risk loci that, taken alone, are neither necessary nor sufficient to cause AD and are thus part of a non-Mendelian, multifactorial etiology. The best known of these is the ApoE4 variant of the apolipoprotein E (ApoE) gene on chromosome 19, which has an unusually large effect size for a common variant. Between 40% and 80% of all individuals with AD have at least one copy of the ApoE4 variant, and the risk for AD in ApoE4 carriers is considerable: a threefold increase for those with a single copy of this risk allele and a 15-fold increase for those with two copies. Ten other candidate risk genes have recently been identified by genome-wide association studies (GWAS), and they are involved in cholesterol metabolism and immune response (Sullivan, Daly, & O'Donovan, 2012).

AD is defined neuropathologically and was first described over 100 years ago by Alois Alzheimer in Germany in 1906. He dissected the brain of a woman who died of dementia in her early 50s after progressive memory impairment that began several years earlier. Alzheimer found numerous neurofibrillary tangles and amyloid plaques in and around the neurons of her neocortex, as well as marked cerebral atrophy. It has since been learned that there is marked loss of both synapses and neurons in

AD and that abnormal proteins are found in both the tangles and plaques. There are also dramatic losses of acetylcholine in AD; the MTL memory structures receive a strong cholinergic input from basal forebrain nuclei. So, a loss of this neurotransmitter could lead to neuronal death. But a cholinergic hypothesis of the cause of AD has lost favor because of the failure of cholinergic agonists to halt or reverse the progression of the disease. So the current focus is on the possible causal role of tangles and plaques.

Intracellular neurofibrillary tangles are composed of twisted filaments of a hyperphosphorylated form of the normal protein tau, which normally acts to stabilize microtubules in the neuron's cytoskeleton. The extracellular plaques have a core of abnormal amyloid beta proteins surrounded by a shell of abnormally shaped fragments of dendrites and axons. One form of amyloid consists of fibrils that are cytotoxic. AD is a protein folding disease (as are prion diseases like "mad cow" disease) in which the cytotoxic forms of both tau and amyloid are abnormally folded.

The causal puzzle is whether the abnormal amyloid (Hardy & Selkoe, 2002) or tau (Maccioni, Farias, Morales, & Navarrete, 2010) comes first in the progression of the disease and how (and whether) each abnormal feature contributes to the death of neurons. Does tau kill neurons whose fragments form the shell of plaques, or does amyloid kill neurons, leading them to fill up with tau? Or could it be both? These two competing, single-cause theories are humorously called the "tau-ist" and "ba-ptist" theories. The letters "ba" in the term "ba-ptist" refer to beta amyloid. From the perspective of a naive outsider, it makes sense that the intracellular process should precede the extracellular one. But the genetic findings would appear to support the amyloid hypothesis, meaning that something about amyloid is cytotoxic and initiates the abnormal intracellular process involving tau. On the other hand, the location of neurofibrillary tangles better tracks the progression of the disease in the brain from its beginning in the MTL to its eventual spread to secondary and tertiary association areas in the neocortex, whereas amyloid plaques have a diffuse distribution in the neocortex (Boller & Duyckaerts, 2003). More recent results have indicated that abnormal protein folding may underlie both key anatomic features of AD, amyloid plaques and neurofibrillary tangles. Abnormal protein folding was first identified in prion-based brain diseases, like mad cow disease, but now appears to be a more general feature of many neurodegenerative diseases. Likewise, any successful explanation of AD will also have to account for the role of neuroinflammation, which is likewise implicated in other neurodegenerative diseases. Such inflammation could be provoked by the abnormal proteins or by the efforts of the immune system to dispose of dead neurons.

So the reader can appreciate that it is very hard to decide between the competing tau and amyloid hypotheses, despite intensive study over several decades. It is sobering for students of behaviorally defined disorders to find that a disorder with a well-defined neuropathology is still unexplained after more than 100 years. There are several reasons why the cause of AD (and by extension many other disorders in this book) is still unknown. The critical events are happening at a molecular level, cannot be observed in real time, and involve many molecular pathways that are not yet fully understood. Regardless of which hypothesis for the cause of AD is correct, we do know that the molecular pathology leads to the death of neurons. And their death eventually leads to brain atrophy that becomes increasingly observable at the macro level as "knife-edge" gyri, wide and deep sulci, and enlarged ventricles. The degree and location of atrophy are closely related to the severity and nature of neuropsychological impairment.

As implied earlier, the neuropsychological hallmark of AD is an initial anterograde amnesia, which appears first in the course of the disease and is caused by the death of neurons in the hippocampus and related structures. However, as the disease progresses to affect other cortical regions, the amnesia in AD becomes broader than MTL amnesia (described in Chapter 9) because it eventually produces a severe retrograde amnesia with confabulated recall (presumably because of frontal lobe involvement). It also produces impairments in aspects of implicit memory (i.e., improved performance on previously encountered perceptual stimuli without conscious recognition of those stimuli) that depend on the neocortex, rather than the basal ganglia (BG). These impaired aspects of implicit memory can be explained by atrophy in posterior cortical regions that contain memory representations for perceptual objects like printed words. In contrast, procedural memory (mediated by the BG) is relatively preserved in AD (but impaired in subcortical dementias, such as PD). Nonamnesic deficits such as aphasia and visuospatial problems are also characteristic of AD, consistent with atrophy of the perisylvian language region and parietal cortex, respectively. Some personality changes are found in AD, although not as extreme as those found in the other dementias considered next.

Frontotemporal Dementia

Frontotemporal dementia (FTD) is the second most common degenerative dementia after AD. FTD is not a single disease, but a family of diseases with similar neuropathology. FTD accounts for about 15–20% of degenerative dementias, whereas AD accounts for more than 50%. The average age of onset of FTD is in the middle 50s and hence younger than in AD. The first clinical symptoms of FTD are dramatic changes in personality rather than cognition, whereas the opposite is true for AD. These personality changes include several that overlap with the orbitofrontal syndrome discussed in Chapter 10 and include lack of inhibition (e.g., swearing, grabbing another's food, sexually inappropriate behavior, and eventually incontinence), lack of empathy, poor grooming, and emotional lability. Patients with FTD also exhibit repetitive, routinized behavior.

The gross neuropathology of FTD includes marked, selective atrophy of frontal and temporal lobes (hence, the name FTD). In this respect, FTD is another cortical dementia, although some types of FTD include subcortical pathology. At a molecular level, FTD is considered to be a tauopathy because neurofibrillary tangles are found in the brains of patients with FTD. In contrast to AD, FTD is not characterized by amyloid plaques. FTD is more familial than AD, but not all of its genetic causes are known. One causal gene variant has been identified on chromosome 17 in the gene for the tau protein.

Subcortical Dementias

In contrast to AD and FTD, which are considered to be cortical dementias, there are subcortical dementias where the main neuropathology is in the BG and other subcortical structures. We have already described one subcortical dementia, PD, in an earlier chapter. About 30% of patients with PD develop dementia. Another subcortical dementia is Huntington's disease (HD), which is a rare autosomal-dominant, single-gene disorder caused by a mutation in a gene on chromosome 4. As in FXS, this gene is disrupted by repetitive sequences of three nucleotides (CAG in HD). So like FXS, HD exhibits anticipation, meaning that the disease becomes more severe (and has an earlier age of onset) across successive generations as the number of repetitive sequences builds up. The mutation in HD is fully penetrant, meaning that every individual who inherits the mutation will get the disease, which invariably produces dementia and eventual death.

At the level of neuropsychology, both PD and HD contrast with AD in having impaired procedural memory (because of impairment in the BG) but less impaired episodic memory (because the hippocampus is relatively spared). Deficits in executive functions and in motor function are prominent in both PD and HD.

CHAPTER SUMMARY

We have reviewed the two main kinds of global disorders, ID syndromes and dementia syndromes. Moderate to severe acquired brain injury can also lead to a global cognitive disorder, and repeated subconcussive events, as are encountered in sports like boxing and football, can lead to a later progressive dementia (CTE). Interestingly, there are some connections between global disorders occurring in childhood (e.g., DS) and dementias that occur in aging (e.g., Alzheimer's disease), and these connections have helped increase our molecular understanding of these disorders. We are closer to providing a multilevel explanation of these global disorders, one that runs from genetic risk factors to neuropathology to neuropsychology to behavior, than we are for most other disorders considered in this book.

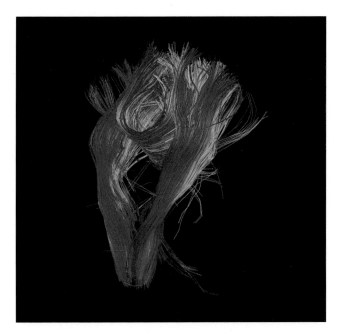

PLATE 5.1. White matter fibers, brainstem, and corpus callosum. White matter fiber architecture of the corpus callosum and brainstem. Measured from diffusion spectral imaging (DSI). The fibers are color-coded by direction: red = left–right, green = anterior–posterior, blue = through brainstem. From *www.humanconnectomeproject.org*. Copyright by the UCLA Laboratory of Neuro Imaging. Reprinted by permission.

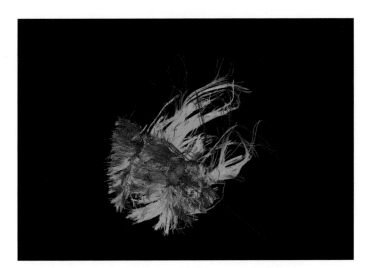

PLATE 10.1. White matter fiber architecture of the prefrontal cortex. Note the longitudinal fibers extending to distant brain structures. Measured from diffusion spectral imaging (DSI). The fibers are color-coded by direction: red = left–right, green = anterior–posterior, blue = through brainstem. From *www.humanconnectomeproject.org*. Copyright by the UCLA Laboratory of Neuro Imaging. Reprinted by permission.

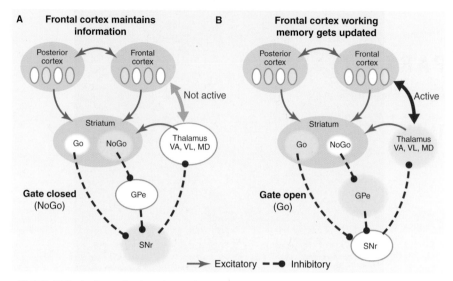

PLATE 10.2. Action selection Go and NoGo pathways involving the basal ganglia and prefrontal cortex. (A) In the default state of no BG activity, or NoGo (indirect) pathway firing in the striatum, the PFC continues to maintain information in an active state. (B) Go (direct) pathway firing triggers updating of a PFC stripe to encode new information. From O'Reilly, Munakata, Frank, Hazy, and Contributors (2012). Copyright 2012 by R. C. O'Reilly and Y. Munakata. Reprinted by permission.

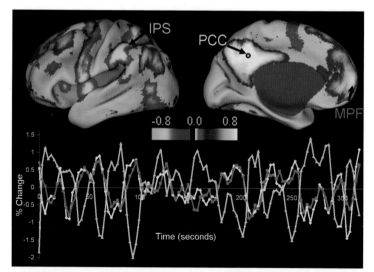

PLATE 13.1. Intrinsic correlations between a seed region in the posterior cingulate cortex (PCC) and all other voxels in the brain for a single subject during resting fixation. The area immediately surrounding the PCC is positively correlated, while the intraparietal sulcus (IPS) is negatively correlated. Below, the time course for a single run is shown for the seed region (PCC; yellow), a region positively correlated with the seed region in the MPF (orange), and a region negatively correlated with the seed region in the IPS (blue). From Fox et al. (2005, p. 9674). Copyright 2005 by the National Academy of Sciences. Reprinted by permission.

PART III

WHAT BECOMES OF THE SELF?

CHAPTER 13

How to Relate Self to Brain

Poor soul the center of my sinful earth,
Rebuke these rebel powers that thee array.
                    —SHAKESPEARE (Sonnet 146)

In this last section of the book, I consider how the brain constructs a self. This topic has been touched on in various ways in previous chapters, but I will draw some of those strands together here with recent neuroscience research that has not been covered previously. As discussed earlier, materialism is incompatible with an immaterial soul, spirit, or mind, and all three of these terms overlap with what can be meant by the term "self." The opening quote from Shakespeare invokes an immaterial soul at war with a material body; this dualistic notion of the relation between soul and body can be traced to Plato and is a dominant idea in Christian theology.

Because of its historical commitment to materialism, much of neuroscience has proceeded without considering the self, partly because the concepts of soul and self have been so similar in Western thought. A second reason for banishing the self from neuroscience is that the concept of self readily becomes a homunculus, and we have seen that explanations in terms of a homunculus do not work because they just postpone the explanatory problem. Having posited a mental homunculus, we still have to explain how it works in material, nonhomuncular terms. A third reason for not considering the self in neuroscience is that the self in everyday thinking is the center of consciousness, the subject of experiences.

Because the problems of consciousness and subjective experience have been considered impossible topics for empirical investigations, neuroscience has avoided considering them until recently. Finally, the concept of a self in much of Western thought has been essentialist: There is *one* self that captures the essence of who we are. This notion of one essential self is captured in Shakespeare's metaphor that the soul is the single center of the bodily earth.

Gillihan and Farah (2005) critically reviewed the neuroimaging literature for differential processing of the self by the brain. They considered two key issues: (1) the essentialist hypothesis that there is a single self (and hence a single center of self in the brain), and (2) whether brain processing differed when self versus non-self was the stimulus in a variety of tasks. They were able to clearly reject the essentialist hypothesis because self-processing occurred in different parts of the brain depending on which task the subject was performing. With regard to the second question, they found some limited evidence that self-processing differed from non-self processing. Their review did not consider the recently discovered default mode network (DMN), discussed later.

A very different perspective on the self in neuroscience comes from the contemporary German philosopher Thomas Metzinger. Metzinger has published two books, *Being No One* (2003) and *The Ego Tunnel* (2009), which describe what he calls the "phenomenal self model" (PSM) constructed by our brain. The first book is written for other philosophers and neuroscientists. The second book explains his theory for a popular audience. The provocative title of his first book refers to a denial of the existence of the essential and substantive self that has dominated Western thought for centuries. Metzinger claims that "nobody ever had or was a self." Instead, humans, and likely certain other animals, have a PSM that is produced by an ongoing brain process that is interrupted by deep sleep and "rebooted" when we awaken. Metzinger argues that the PSM provides a transparent interface with both the external world and our interoceptive states, transparent because we are not aware of the cognitive and neural mechanisms that produce the PSM; we are only aware of its constructed contents. Consistent with the "information integration theory of consciousness" (Tononi, 2004), the PSM provides a coherent self-representation for global cognitive control.

Metzinger and his colleagues have explored the PSM with empirical studies of phenomena like the rubber hand illusion, described earlier, and a more dramatic whole-body illusion. In the latter illusion, participants see a three-dimensional image (or avatar) of themselves from the rear projected several feet ahead of them, while their actual back is being stroked at the same time they see their projected back being stroked. After about a minute of stroking, participants feel their bodily self "jump" into the self avatar in front of them. In other words, the anomalous input is resolved by an out-of-body experience.

Metzinger (2003) argues that these and other self-illusions, such as those discussed in this book (e.g., phantoms, synesthesia, alien hand, prosopagnosia, delusion and hallucinations in schizophrenia, and denial of blindness), reveal that the typical PSM is a construction or simulation that can be selectively disrupted. Ironically, despite his claim that traditional selves do not exist, Metzinger (2003) has mustered some of the most compelling arguments and evidence for why we cannot ignore the self in human neuroscience.

In what follows, I will present three other arguments for why we cannot dispense with the self in neuroscience and the evidence that supports them. The first argument is based on biology; the second considers multiple forms of self-knowledge, consistent with Gillihan and Farah's (2005) rejection of the essentialist hypothesis of self; and the third is recent compelling evidence for distinct self-processing in the DMN.

THE SELF IS DEEPLY BIOLOGICAL

The distinction between self and non-self is deeply biological, so perhaps we can make some headway on how the self is represented in the nervous system without diving headlong into the problem of consciousness. Making such headway is possible because the self exists in the body outside of the nervous system and outside of consciousness. Indeed, conscious self-representations are a very recent evolutionary achievement, but one that builds on much older ones.

To survive, any organism, whether a single cell, a plant, or a vertebrate animal, has to have a boundary between self- and non-self and carefully regulate what things are allowed to cross that boundary. A physical boundary is needed because all living things are *islands against entropy*. By this phrase, I mean that living things (temporarily) break the second law of thermodynamics, which states that all matter tends toward less organized and less energetic states. Living things are able to violate the second law because they have a free source of energy, basically our sun. The basic unit of selection in evolution (with some possible exceptions that are not important here) is the individual organism. Natural selection favored individual organisms that (1) better utilized this free energy to build ever more complex structures inside themselves, and (2) better protected their interior from harmful aspects of the external environment. These harmful aspects of the external environment are constantly threatening to enforce the second law and reduce any living thing back to individual atoms and molecules. If there is too much or too little heat, water, or oxygen, too many or too few ions or nutrients in the external environment, the organism is doomed. So, maintaining homeostasis is a basic life function for any living thing, from a single cell to a human being, and the mechanisms for maintaining homeostasis had to evolve as organisms became more complex. Similarly, boundaries evolved for protecting self from non-self. The most basic boundary used by living things is the cell membrane, and this boundary is maintained in multicellular organisms like ourselves who have evolved other boundaries, such as the skin.

Another example of how the distinction between self and non-self is deeply biological is the immune system. Organisms need protection not only from the nonliving, inorganic environment, but also from other organisms and the organic molecules they produce. The immune system is exquisitely "designed" to distinguish self from non-self at the molecular level and to rapidly deploy defensive mechanisms not only to eliminate foreign molecules, but also to "remember" them so they can be eliminated more quickly in the future. There are many interesting parallels between the immune system and the nervous system, as well as an important relation between them, but that is a topic for another time.

So, it should not be at all surprising that the evolution of nervous systems maintained and enhanced the deeply biological distinction between self and non-self. It had to maintain this distinction in order to enable basic survival goals by allowing higher levels of control over basic homeostatic processes. As discussed in Chapter 11, the ANS and the CNS structures that regulate it (such as the hypothalamus) maintain homeostasis in humans and other vertebrates, and much of this homeostasis proceeds unconsciously. As levels of the CNS higher than the hypothalamus evolved, and thus higher levels of control of homeostasis, the distinction between self and non-self was necessarily maintained because the unit of selection continued to be the individual organism.

MULTIPLE ASPECTS OF THE SELF IN THE BRAIN

Consequently, we should not expect a single self-representation in the CNS, but it is reasonable to expect different aspects of self to be represented and processed in different parts of the CNS. A prescient statement of this view was elaborated by Neisser (1988), who distinguished five kinds of self-knowledge, which we can relate to different parts of the brain. These five kinds are (1) the ecological self, (2) the **interpersonal self**, (3) the extended or **autobiographical self**, (4) the private self, and (5) the conceptual self. The preceding chapters have reviewed the brain systems involved in most of these kinds of self-knowledge. Perhaps we should say "self-representation" instead of "self-knowledge" to allow for implicit, nonconscious self processes.

As we have seen in Chapter 6, the *ecological* or **bodily self** is represented in the primary and secondary somatosensory cortex, which processes the body schema and its relation to the external world. We have also discussed pathologies of this body schema, including phantom limbs and neglect of one half of the body. In these contrasting pathologies, an absent limb is sensed as present (a phantom) versus a present limb being treated as absent (neglect). Both pathologies demonstrate that our seemingly direct and immediate knowledge of our body is constructed by the brain and can be selectively disrupted, with a consequent change in the conscious self-representation.

The *interpersonal* self was discussed in Chapter 11, where we described how intersubjectivity develops and which parts of the brain are activated by theory of mind tasks. As discussed in that chapter, there has been considerable neuroscience work on this aspect of self since Neisser's (1988) article. In autism spectrum disorder, the interpersonal self does not develop properly, leading to a profound change in conscious experience.

The *extended* or *autobiographical* self was discussed in Chapter 9, where we saw how episodic memories are consolidated by the hippocampal complex, and how amnesias resulting from damage to the hippocampus and related structures disrupt the autobiographical self. We also reviewed recent work demonstrating that the hippocampus is important for episodic imagery, such as imagining a future event.

The brain structures supporting a *private*, or we could say **interoceptive self**, were discussed in Chapter 11 and involve a hierarchy of midline structures. The explosion of research in affective neuroscience has greatly changed what we know about this part of self in the brain. Psychoanalysts have long theorized that emotions form the core of the self, and developmentalists have documented the role of emotional exchanges in the infant's development of a self (e.g., Stern, 1985). Affective neuroscience has now provided us with a much deeper understanding of how this affective core of the self is realized in the brain (Damasio, 2010; Panksepp & Biven, 2012). Disorders of state regulation, such as major depressive disorder (MDD) or bipolar disorder (BPD), can alter the conscious, private self-representation so that it becomes fixated on painful or euphoric states. While we have empathy for someone with such a disorder, we cannot fully feel what it is like to be them unless we have had the disorder ourselves.

Finally, there is the *conceptual* self, which consists of all the beliefs, roles, and attributes a person would endorse as belonging to them (i.e., their self-concept). It is the conceptual self that psychology has traditionally been most concerned with, and that at first blush seems harder to relate to the brain, partly because it draws on the previous four kinds of self. But some recent developments in neuroscience suggest some brain areas may preferentially activate something like a conceptual self in certain situations. We will discuss this recent work next when we talk about the DMN.

There are also important aspects of the self discussed in the previous chapters that do not fall readily under Neisser's (1988) five categories. Chief among these are action selection and action monitoring, both discussed in Chapter 10. For example, the intentional self is altered in schizophrenia in a way that leads to striking errors in the attribution of thoughts and action.

THE DEFAULT MODE NETWORK AND SELF-PROCESSING IN THE BRAIN

An important and fairly recent discovery is that there is a network of brain sites that is activated when individuals are supposedly "at rest" and whose activity is anticorrelated with the activity of other networks prompted by various cognitive tasks. This **default mode network (DMN)** was discovered by Raichle and colleagues about a decade ago (e.g., Gusnard & Raichle, 2001) and has since been an important focus of research in both typical individuals and those with disorders. A variety of lines of evidence has shown that DMN activity reflects thinking about the self: what we label in common parlance as daydreaming, worrying, remembering, and planning. So, the mind at rest is actually very busy. All of us at times find it hard to focus on external tasks because we are so preoccupied with the internal ones. As we will see below, this internal focus is exaggerated in a number of psychopathologies (see Whitfield-Gabrieli & Ford, 2012, for a review).

Prior to the discovery of the DMN, it had long been known that the resting brain is metabolically active, as demonstrated by the discovery of the resting EEG (Berger, 1929), and by the hyperfrontality of the resting brain found in early regional cerebral blood flow (rCBF) studies (Ingvar, 1979). But neither of these imaging approaches could localize the network of brain structures that were, as it turned out, selectively active at rest. Nor could early imaging examine the relation of these at-rest networks to the other networks that are activated by externally prompted behavioral tasks. The use of fMRI methods accomplished both of these goals (Raichle et al., 2001) and later demonstrated functional connectivity among the hubs in the DMN, distinct from the functional connectivity among hubs characterizing other networks (Greicius et al., 2007). Another important discovery about the DMN was that its activity is "turned down" when other task-relevant networks are "turned on" (see Plate 13.1 in the color insert). So stimulus-independent thought (supported by the DMN) alternates with, and is in competition with, stimulus- or task-dependent thought. Moreover, the degree of anticorrelation between DMN activity and task-relevant network activity was found to be related to task performance. Greater anticorrelation predicted better task performance, as would be expected given that we have limited attentional resources and thus need to allocate them to the task at hand. We all know from firsthand experience that we do not work as well when we are preoccupied.

So, what happens if we cannot switch off the DMN, even when it is adaptive to do so? One can readily imagine that DMN "malfunction" occurring in a variety of psychopathologies; Whitfield-Gabrieli and Ford (2012) review the evidence for altered DMN activity in schizophrenia and mood disorders, and mention that DMN abnormalities are also found in ADHD and autism. The key question, of course, is whether DMN activity differences in these disorders are part of the *cause* of these disorders or just a *consequence* of them. If causal, other factors will be needed to explain why these disorders are distinct.

CHAPTER SUMMARY

We can view recent work on the neuroscience of the self as a sign that by analyzing the parts of the human brain, we have discovered enough about how it works to move on to the process of reconstructing it. In science, breaking down a phenomenon into its relevant parts precedes studies of how those parts interact: analysis precedes synthesis. For phenomena that arise in a complex system like the human brain, the phenomena can only be explained as emergent properties of the interactions among the parts.

The PSM is an important emergent property of the interactions among the parts of the brain, one that is distorted in characteristic ways in the various disorders of abnormal behavior that we have considered in this book. So, neuroscience is now embarking on the second half of the round trip envisioned at the beginning of the book in Figure 1.1, which is reconstructing our mental experience. Since this is a new direction, we can expect that many new insights lie ahead in our quest to understand both normal and abnormal behavior.

APPENDIX A

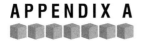

Human Neocortical Regions

	Names	Brodmann's area	Some associated functions
	SENSATION, PERCEPTION, MOTOR		
Visual	Primary visual cortex (striate cortex).	17	Retinoptic map, basic visual features
	Secondary visual cortex (extrastriate cortex)	18, 19	Higher-level features (e.g., color, motion)
Auditory	Primary auditory cortex (Heschl's gyrus)	41, 42	Tonotopic map, basic auditory features
	Secondary auditory cortex (superior temporal gyrus [STG])	22	Higher-level features (e.g., phonemes)
Somatosensory	Primary somatosensory cortex (postcentral gyrus)	1, 2, 3	Somatotopic map, basic somesthetic features
	Secondary somatosensory cortex	5, 7 (rostral)	Higher-level features (e.g., tactile perception)

	Names	Brodmann's area	Some associated functions
SENSATION, PERCEPTION, MOTOR *(continued)*			
Motor	Primary motor cortex	4	Motor homunculus, simple movements
	Secondary motor cortex (supplementary motor area [SMA])	6	Basic-movement planning
	Frontal eye fields (FEFs)	8	Eye-movement control
	Broca's area	44, 45	Mouth-movement control
INTEGRATION			
Posterior	Angular gyrus (AG)	39	Reading, language, math
	Superior parietal lobule (SPL) (medial portion is precuneus)	7	Spatial orientation
	Supramarginal gyrus (SMG)	40	Language processing
	Superior temporal sulcus (STS)	—	Social and speech perception
	Middle temporal gyrus (MTG)	21	Language processing
	Inferior temporal gyrus	20	Face and object perception
	Fusiform gyrus	37	Face and object perception
	Temporal pole (TP)	38	Domain-general semantic knowledge, self-information
Posterior medial	Posterior cingulate gyrus (PCG)	23, 26, 29, 30, 31	Default mode network (DMN)
	Parahippocampal gyrus (PHG)	27, 28, 34, 35, 36	Memory encoding and retrieval

	Names	Brodmann's area	Some associated functions
	INTEGRATION *(continued)*		
Anterior lateral	Dorsolateral prefrontal cortex (DLPFC)	9, 46	Working memory
	Frontal pole (FP)	10	Abstract planning
	Orbitofrontal cortex (OFC)	11, 12, 47	Affective decision making
Anterior medial	Dorsal anterior	32	Default mode network (DMN)
	Anterior cingulate gyrus (ACG)	24, 33	Error detection and conflict monitoring
	Subgenual cingulate gyrus (SCG)	25	Hub for state regulation

APPENDIX B
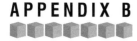

Online Resources

Digital Anatomist Project
User-friendly software to learn human anatomy, including neuroanatomy.
http://da.biostr.washington.edu/da.html

Brain Factors.org
A public information initiative cosponsored by the Society for Neuroscience to share scientific knowledge about the brain and mind and to dispel "neuro-myths."

Neurosynth
Provides meta-analyses of human fMRI studies.
http://neurosynth.org

The Human Connectome Project
Provides meta-analyses of structural and functional connectivity of the human brain.
www.humanconnectomeproject.org

Computational Cognitive Neuroscience (2012) by R. C. O'Reilly
    and Y. Munakata
Online Wiki textbook that explains neural network models of human brain functions and provides links to simulation projects that allow the student to run neural network demonstrations.
http://grey.colorado.edu/CompCogNeuro/index.php/CCNBook/Main

Online Mendelian Inheritance in Man (OMIM)

Comprehensive data on human genes and their functions.

www.ncbi.nlm.nih.gov/omim

Encyclopedia of DNA Elements (ENCODE)

A public research consortium that is analyzing all the functional elements in the human genome, which include regulatory elements involved in epigenesis.

www.genome.gov

Glossary

Achromotopsia—absence of color vision, either acquired (due to a brain lesion in visual cortex) or congenital (due to genetic variation that affects neurons in the retina that process color).

Agnosia—literally, "without knowledge"; agnosia is a neurological syndrome in which there is an impairment in perceptual recognition ability within a sensory modality, such as vision or audition, or even for a particular class of objects (e.g., human faces or voices) without an elementary sensory deficit or reduced level of alertness.

Akinetopsia—loss of motion perception caused by an acquired brain lesion in visual cortex.

Alertness and arousal—the most basic attentional state, which is absent in deep sleep, coma, and even some waking states, such as a persistent vegetative state or a minimally conscious state.

Alien-hand syndrome—a rare neurological syndrome, usually associated with damage to the corpus callosum and medial frontal cortex, in which the patient's hand makes meaningful movements that the patient does not experience as intended.

Amygdala—almond-shaped nuclei located adjacent to the hippocampus deep within the medial temporal lobes of the brain in complex vertebrates, including humans. The amygdala plays a major role in emotional reactions and conditioning, especially for fear.

Anisometry hypothesis—an explanation of attentional neglect (see below), which holds that the perceptual representation of external space is itself distorted so as to be asymmetric. The biased competition model (see below) offers a competing explanation of neglect.

Aphasias—neurological syndromes in which aspects of spoken language are disrupted without there being a sensory or motor deficit to explain the symptoms.

Apperceptive agnosia—a subtype of agnosia (usually visual) in which elementary sensory processing is intact, but there is an inability to bind basic perceptual features into a meaningful whole. A patient with this subtype of visual agnosia cannot draw visual objects or say whether two visual objects are alike and has difficulty recognizing them, especially when the orientation is unusual or the image is degraded.

Arcuate fasciculus—an intrahemispheric white matter tract that connects posterior neocortex with anterior neocortex, including Wernicke's area in the left temporal lobe and Broca's area in the left frontal lobe. Consequently, the left hemisphere arcuate fasciculus is important in language processing.

Associative agnosia—another subtype of agnosia (usually visual) in which perceptual binding of features is intact, but semantic significance of the object is unavailable. A patient with this subtype of visual agnosia can draw visual objects but has trouble identifying the function or typical location of the object.

Attentional neglect—a neurological syndrome in which there is failure of awareness of stimuli in the side of space opposite to a unilateral brain lesion that cannot be accounted for by elementary motor or sensory problems.

Autobiographical self—the aspect of self-representation that includes one's past and one's imagined futures.

Autonomic nervous system (ANS)—the part of the nervous system that is involved in automatic homeostatic regulation of basic bodily functions, such as heart rate, breathing, digestion, and neuroendocrine functions. The ANS bridges the central and peripheral nervous systems; peripheral portions include the sympathetic, parasympathetic, and enteric (gastrointestinal) branches. The central portions include the amygdala and hypothalamus, with the latter controlling neuroendocrine functions.

Bálint syndrome—a neurological syndrome following a bilateral posterior brain lesion that produces a severe form of attentional neglect in which awareness is limited to a single object at a time. *See* Simultagnosia.

Biased-competition model—an explanation of hemineglect, which posits that acquired brain damage produces an imbalance in attentional control between the two cerebral hemispheres, which certain treatments can partly alleviate. This model contrasts with a subtraction model in which one attentional field is eliminated and cannot be restored.

Binocular rivalry—a perceptual phenomenon that is elicited by presenting two different visual stimuli to each eye. Instead of fusing the two visual inputs into one image, the viewer experiences alternation between one image and the other.

Blindsight—the preservation of low-level, implicit visual detection in cortical blindness without explicit visual experience.

Bodily self—the aspect of self-representation that includes one's own body.

Broca's aphasia—a subtype of aphasia characterized by impaired speech fluency (speech is halting and telegraphic).

Chromotopsia—a neurological syndrome following acquired damage in which only color but not form is perceived; hence, it is the opposite of cortical achromotopsia.

Classical conditioning—a basic form of learning in which an unconditioned response (e.g., salivating to food or an eye blink to a puff of air) becomes associated with an arbitrary stimulus (e.g., a tone or a color) such that this conditioned stimulus is sufficient to produce the response by itself. It is also called Pavlovian conditioning after the scientist who discovered it.

Cognitive-map theory—E. C. Tolman's theory that animals in a conditioning study form mental representations of the spatial environment that allow them to make novel predictions about where a reward will be found. By demonstrating that stimulus–response associations alone could not account for an animal's behavior, Tolman posed a severe challenge to behaviorism.

Conduction aphasia—a subtype of aphasia proposed by Carl Wernicke in which disconnection of the white matter pathway (arcuate fasciculus) between the two main neocortical language centers (Broca's area and Wernicke's area), rather than damage to these language centers themselves, caused a characteristic profile of impaired and intact language functions: intact fluency (unlike Broca's aphasia) and intact comprehension (unlike Wernicke's aphasia), but impaired repetition of speech.

Confabulation—"honest lying," confabulation is a narrative constructed by a patient with brain damage relying on partial information. An outside observer can readily see the narrative is false.

Consilience—a term proposed by E. O. Wilson for the principle that evidence from independent, unrelated sources can "converge" to yield strong conclusions. The consilience principle is related to the network theory of scientific truth, in which any aspect of current scientific knowledge constrains potential explanations for novel phenomena.

Convergence zone—a portion of the brain with inputs from many other brain areas. Two key convergence zones are the hippocampal formation and the prefrontal cortex.

Corollary discharge—a copy of a motor command sent to sensory portions of the brain so they will disregard changes in sensory input caused by the organism's own movement; also called an *efference copy*.

Declarative long-term memory—a form of long-term memory for knowledge that can be declared, including both semantic knowledge, such as people's names, word spellings, and definitions, and episodic knowledge of discrete events in one's own life.

Declarative theory—a theory of the function of the hippocampus in long-term memory proposed by Larry R. Squire, which holds that an intact hippocampus is necessary for the acquisition of both semantic *and* episodic knowledge.

Deep dyslexia—a subtype of acquired dyslexia in which the patient cannot read non-words and makes semantic errors when reading real words (e.g., reading "ship" when presented with the written word "yacht").

Default mode network (DMN)—one of several resting state functional networks in the brain, the DMN involves medial cortical structures (principally the medial prefrontal cortex and the precuneus) and mediates thoughts about the self when one is at rest. The activity of the DMN is negatively correlated with the activity of other functional networks involved in externally prompted cognitive tasks.

Disconnection—a model for explaining abnormal behavior first proposed by Carl Wernicke in which damage to the connection between cortical processing centers disrupts function, rather than damage to the center itself. *See also* Conduction aphasia.

Discourse—the linking of sentences such that they constitute a narrative.

Distal object—in the science of perception, an object in the external world whose physical signal is detected by sensory organs in the brain to produce a proximal stimulus.

Dorsal visual pathway—a visual pathway specialized for "where" and "how" information (spatial reference frames) that passes through the parietal lobes. *See also* Ventral visual pathway.

Double dissociation—two opposite dissociations of abilities in two patient groups: group A is selectively impaired on ability X, whereas group B is selectively impaired on ability Y. Double dissociations in neuropsychology argue for the independence of two abilities, but this approach faces significant criticisms.

Dual-process theory—a theory of printed word recognition proposed by Max Coltheart in which there are two routes for pronouncing a printed word, a direct and an indirect route. The direct route matches the abstract sequence of graphemes in the printed word to an entry for that word in the mental lexicon. The indirect route uses grapheme–phoneme correspondence rules to derive the pronunciation of the printed word.

Dysarthria—Problems in speech production caused by damaged motor pathways in the articulatory system. Dysarthria is distinct from aphasia.

Dyspraxia—inability to program motor sequences in the absence of a basic motor deficit. Dyspraxia can affect different motor outputs, mainly articulatory gestures (speech dyspraxia) or functional limb movements (ideomotor dyspraxia).

Echoic memory—very brief, short-term sensory memory for sounds.

Efference copy—*see* Corollary discharge.

Élan vital—French for "life force," this term is from a dualist theory of life called vitalism. In this theory, matter could be alive only if it was infused with the life force. Biology was able to disprove vitalism.

Emergent properties—new properties in a system that are not strictly reducible to individual elements of that system. For instance, water (H_2O), a liquid, has physical and chemical properties that are quite distinct from the properties of either hydrogen or oxygen, both gases, which are the two elements that combine to make water. Another example is provided by isomers, organic molecules with identical chemical compositions but different structures (e.g., mirror images of each other), which affect their interaction with other molecules.

Empiricism—in philosophy, the view that all human knowledge derives from experience. The contrasting view, *idealism*, holds that at least some knowledge precedes experience.

Engram—a term coined by Karl Lashley that means the neural representation of a specific memory. Lashley discovered from lesion studies that engrams were not localized to a particular part of the brain.

Enteric nervous system—a part of the ANS in the gastrointestinal tract that controls digestion. *See* Autonomic nervous system (ANS).

Environmental dependency—a neurological symptom observed after damage to the frontal lobes in which the patient's behavior is driven by the immediate context, regardless of whether the behavior is appropriate. Also called "stimulus-bound" behavior or "capture errors" in typical individuals without brain damage.

Epigenesis—(1) literally, "upon formation"; epigenesis is a theory of how the forms of living organisms arise that was first articulated by Aristotle. Epigenesis holds that form emerges as a result of a developmental process and is not preexistent in the fertilized egg. *See* Preformation theory for the opposite theory. (2) literally, "above the genes"; epigenesis in this second sense is the study of heritable changes in gene expression or cellular phenotype caused by mechanisms other than changes in the underlying DNA sequence.

Episodic imagery—Imagined future episodes of one's life, which are mediated by the hippocampus.

Episodic long-term memory (LTM)—a subtype of declarative long-term memory mediated by the hippocampus that includes memory for events or episodes in one's own life.

Equipotentiality—a term first used by Karl Lashley to describe the distributed nature of storage of new long-term memories in the brain. This term is also used for the ability of a brain structure to take on different functions in development or after a brain lesion. The opposite of equipotentiality would be strict localization of function.

Experience-dependent synaptogenesis—a lifelong mechanism of brain plasticity in which new synapses are formed or eliminated to encode new experiences of the individual animal.

Experience-expectant synaptogenesis—an early, genetically programmed overproduction of synapses in the developing brain that are strengthened or pruned based on experiences that are virtually universal for that species (e.g., visual and auditory input, gravity, faces and voices for human infants).

Explicit long-term memory—another name for declarative long-term memory (see above).

Global aphasia—a subtype of aphasia that combines the characteristics of both Broca's and Wernicke's aphasia.

Grandmother cell hypothesis—the idea that only a single neuron is dedicated to the representation of specific aspects of an individual's knowledge, such as the face of one's grandmother.

Hemineglect—failure to attend to or act in one side of visual space.

Homotopy—a general principle of the organization of primary sensory areas in which the dimensions of a physical stimulus are mapped onto primary sensory cortex. For vision and touch, the spatial dimensions of the external world are mapped onto primary sensory cortex.

Hypothalamus—a small collection of nuclei in the brain that handle homeostatic functions and are part of the central ANS. *See also* Autonomic nervous system (ANS).

Iconic memory—a very brief form of visual short-term memory, similar to *echoic memory*.

Idealism—in philosophy, the theory that ideas are preexistent and innate and are not derived from experience, in contrast to *empiricism*. Idealism is related to nativism, the term more commonly used in psychology to contrast with empiricism.

Implicit long-term memory—nondeclarative long-term memory, consisting of memories that are formed based on repeated experiences and result in changes in behavior but cannot be consciously recalled. Unlike explicit memory, implicit memory does not depend on medial temporal lobe structures.

Imprinting—any kind of phase-sensitive learning (learning occurring at a particular age or a particular life stage) that is rapid and apparently independent of the consequences of behavior. It was first used to describe situations in which an animal or person learns the characteristics of some stimulus, which is therefore said to be "imprinted" onto the subject. Imprinting is hypothesized to have a critical period.

Inhibition of return—an aspect of visual behavior that develops in infancy in which a previously fixated location is unlikely to be fixated again. Inhibition of return is hypothesized to facilitate complete scanning of the environment.

Insula—from the Latin word for island, the insula is a part of cortex found beneath the sylvian fissure on the neocortical surface. It is involved in interoception, the perception of stimuli coming directly from the body, such as pain.

Intentional neglect—a form of hemineglect in which movements to contralesional space are restricted (also called motor neglect), in contrast to sensory or *attentional neglect* (see above).

Interactive activation model—an early neural network model, devised by J. McClelland and D. Rumelhart, in which information flows in both directions, allowing later stages of processing to influence earlier ones. This model accounts for top-down effects in perception.

Interactive specialization—a theory of brain–behavior development proposed by Mark Johnson in which the localization of specific functions develops as a result of a process of interaction among different brain regions. Early in development, more brain regions participate in that function, which then gradually becomes consolidated in a smaller set of brain regions.

Interneurons—neurons in the brain that are not directly connected to sensory inputs or motor outputs, and so are involved in intermediate processing between inputs and outputs. Hence, interneurons are found outside the primary motor cortex and primary sensory cortices and comprise a majority of neurons in the human brain.

Interoceptive self—an aspect of self that represents bodily experiences and emotions; also called the "private self."

Interpersonal self—an aspect of self that represents relations with other people.

Inversion effect—a phenomenon in visual perception of faces in which it is harder to recognize an upside-down face.

Lateral syndrome—one of three neurological syndromes associated with damage to different parts of the prefrontal cortex, or PFC (lateral, medial, and ventral). The lateral syndrome is associated with damage to the dorsolateral PFC, leading to deficits in working memory and novel problem solving. *See also* Medial syndrome and Ventral syndrome.

Lexicon—the mental representation of all the words in an individual's vocabulary for a given language, including each word's pronunciation, meaning, and syntactic function. The lexicon of individuals who know how to read also includes the spelling of all the words they recognize in print.

Locus coeruleus (LC)—literally, the "blue spot"; the LC is a nucleus in the midbrain portion of the brainstem containing neurons that release norepinephrine into widely distributed sites across the whole brain.

Long-term memory (LTM)—memories that, unlike short term memory (STM), last longer than a few minutes and depend on a structural change in brain synapses. LTM can be divided into explicit and implicit LTM, and there are several subtypes of each.

Mass effect—a termed coined by Karl Lashley to describe the effect of experimental lesions on long-term memory in laboratory animals, which Lashley found depended not on their location but on their extent.

Materialism—a core doctrine of modern science which holds that scientific explanations must be based on matter and energy and not on immaterial entities or forces. Materialism is essentially synonymous with *naturalism*, which holds that the province of science is things found in nature, not supernatural things.

Medial syndrome—a neurological syndrome following damage to the medial surface of the prefrontal cortex (PFC) and/or nearby anterior cingulate cortex, in which there is a marked decrease in the initiation of behavior and sometimes a deficit in self-monitoring. A severe form of the medial syndrome is akinetic mutism, in which the patient is conscious but neither moves nor speaks. The medial syndrome is one of three different PFC syndromes. *See also* Lateral syndrome; Ventral syndrome.

Methylation—a mechanism of gene regulation in which methyl (CH3-) groups are attached to the DNA in a gene, preventing the gene from being expressed. Methylation is one mechanism of *epigenesis* (see definition 2 of epigenesis above).

Microcephaly—a developmental disorder in which the brain is abnormally small. Microcephaly is found in several intellectual disability syndromes, such as Down syndrome and Williams syndrome, and may be produced by single gene mutations or environmental teratogens acting during fetal life.

Mind–body problem—a key and contentious puzzle in the philosophy of mind that is concerned with how a physical body (more specifically, a physical brain) gives rise to conscious experience. Numerous solutions to this problem have been proposed in the history of philosophy, but without a satisfying resolution. Cognitive neuroscience is attempting to solve this problem with empirical methods.

Mismatch negativity (MMN)—a phenomenon observed in EEG or MEG recordings in which the brain has a greater response to a slightly different stimulus occurring in a long sequence of identical stimuli. The MMN can be used to determine which stimuli are perceptually distinct for a given group or individual.

Morphemes—the smallest units of meaning in a language, which often corresponds to a single word (e.g., "red") but may be only part of a word (e.g., *un-* in "unlikely").

Motor homunculus—the representation of the body in the primary motor cortex of the brain, with the size of the map of a particular body part corresponding to how many neurons are needed to control its movements. So, the representation of the mouth (in humans) is much larger than the representation of many physically larger body parts.

Multiple memory trace (MMT) theory—a theory of episodic long-term memory formation proposed by Lyn Nadel, which holds that episodic memories never become independent of the hippocampus, in contrast to the consolidation theory, which holds that consolidated episodic memories do not depend on the hippocampus. Instead, the MMT theory holds that each time a given episodic memory is retrieved it is encoded anew in the hippocampus (hence "multiple traces"). The two theories thus make competing predictions about the extent of loss of past episodic memories (retrograde amnesia) after hippocampal damage. MMT predicts much worse retrograde amnesia than does the consolidation theory.

Narcolepsy—a medical syndrome in which the patient abruptly falls asleep, even at inappropriate times (e.g., while driving). Narcolepsy can be caused by damage to sleep regulation circuits in the hypothalamus.

Naturalism—*See* Materialism.

Nonassociative learning—a form of implicit long-term memory in which the level of brain arousal to a stimulus changes, but in which there is not a learned association between a stimulus and an overt motor response. Sensitization and habituation are the main forms of nonassociative learning.

Nondeclarative long-term memory—*See* Implicit long-term memory.

Nondisjunction—failure of paired chromosomes to split apart, nondisjunction is a genetic error that can occur in the process of meiosis, a type of cell division that produces sperm and egg cells (gametes). After each chromosome is copied, *two* copies of a chromosome go to one daughter cell and *no* copy goes to the other daughter cell. Hence, the chromosome number is abnormal in each of the two resulting gamete cells. If such an abnormal gamete is involved in conception, the resulting fetus will have an abnormal chromosome number (i.e., aneuploidy) in every cell in its body. Down syndrome is caused mainly by nondisjunction of chromosome 21.

Nucleus accumbens (NAcc)—the ventral portion of the striatum or basal ganglia in the brain, the NAcc is part of the median forebrain bundle that when stimulated leads to intense seeking behavior. The NAcc is important in normal reward learning and is altered in addicted behaviors.

Obligatory attention—a normal stage of infant visual development in which eye gaze is captured by a stimulus and cannot be readily disengaged.

Orbitofrontal cortex (OFC)—a portion of the prefrontal cortex that lies above the orbits of the eyes, the OFC is an important structure in regulation of emotion and motivation.

Overflow movement—a developmentally normal form of unintended movement in which other parts of the body move when an intended movement is made. Overflow movement is frequent in infancy and toddlerhood, but can occur normally in older individuals during intense effort.

Pavlovian conditioning—*See* Classical conditioning.

Perceptual priming—facilitation of perception of a stimulus following the presentation of a priming stimulus.

Perceptual rivalry—a phenomenon that arises in perception when we are presented with an ambiguous figure, like the Necker cube (Figure 6.4), or two distinct objects, one to each eye. Because the visual input in these cases supports two competing interpretations, our perceptual experience alternates between the two interpretations (instead of fusing them).

Periaqueductal gray matter (PAG)—also called central gray matter, the PAG consists of collections of neurons around the cerebral aqueduct in the tegmentum of the midbrain, which play a role in pain and analgesia and also produce automatic defensive behaviors when stimulated. Damage to the PAG results in loss of consciousness, indicating that PAG is necessary but not sufficient for consciousness.

Peripheral autonomic nervous system (pANS)—*See* Autonomic nervous system (ANS).

Phantom limb pain—the experience of pain in a missing limb, usually one that is lost because of injury, but it has been reported in people with congenital absence of a limb.

Phonemes—an abstract linguistic representation, a phoneme is the smallest difference in sound in a spoken word that signals a difference in meaning (e.g., we
distinguish the two words /bat/ and /pat/, which differ in their initial phoneme
/b/ vs. /p/). Most spoken words contain several phonemes, and individual letters
in an alphabet usually represent individual phonemes.

Precuneus—literally, a brain structure in front of the cuneus (Latin for "wedge,"
the cuneus is Brodmann's area 17 or V1 in the occipital lobe). So, the precuneus
(Brodmann's areas 7 and 31) is a posterior medial structure of the cortex, specifically the medial portion of the superior parietal lobule, located just above the
posterior cingulate gyrus. The precuneus is part of the default mode network. *See
also* Default mode network (DMN).

Preformation theory—*See* Epigenesis, definition 2.

Procedural memory—a form of implicit long-term memory for motor skills, statistical learning, and reward-based learning, mediated by the basal ganglia and
cerebellum. *See also* Implicit memory.

Prosody—the vocal intonation contour of an utterance that can modify the literal
meaning of words and sentences, prosody can convey emotional information.
Unlike structural language, which is mediated mainly by the left hemisphere,
prosody is mediated by the right hemisphere in typical adults.

Prosopagnosia—a selective inability to recognize individual faces despite the ability
to perceive that the stimulus is a face. May occur as a developmental or acquired
disorder.

Protodeclarative gestures—before the advent of spoken language, typical infants
use manual gestures to draw attention to an interesting object in the world. These
gestures have a communicative function that is similar to a spoken declarative
sentence (e.g., "There is a dog.")

Protoimperative gestures—before the advent of spoken language, typical infants
use manual gestures to request desired objects. These gestures have a communicative function that is similar to a spoken imperative (e.g., "Give me the cookie!")

Pure insertion—an assumption in cognitive science that a single stage or component
of processing can be added or subtracted without affecting other stages or components. The *subtraction model* (*see below*) of interpreting the results of brain damage
or neuroimaging studies in typical individuals assumes pure insertion.

Qualia—"raw feels"; qualia are individual instances of subjective, conscious experience.

Raphe nuclei (RN)—a cluster of nuclei found in the brainstem that regulate the
release of serotonin.

Reconstructionism—in science, the opposite of reductionism. Once the essential elements of some aspect of nature (a phenomenon) have been discovered, the next stage in a scientific explanation is to demonstrate how the interactions among those elements produce the phenomenon.

Reductionism—a method for explaining a complex phenomenon by breaking it up into component parts. The first phase of any scientific investigation involves reduction. So, a chemical like water (H^2O) can be reduced to the elements of hydrogen and oxygen. A full explanation of a complex phenomenon often requires demonstrating how the interactions among component parts produce the phenomenon in question. *See also* Emergent properties.

Reticular activating system (RAS)—part of the brain, originating in the brainstem, that is involved in alertness and arousal and sleep.

Retinotopic—homotopic mapping of the inputs to the retina onto the thalamus and primary visual cortex.

Reverse inference—in functional neuroimaging research, studies which use patterns of brain activation to predict the behavior subjects were engaged in during the scan.

Selective attention—one of several forms of attention, characterized by focusing on a few things (sensory inputs, thoughts, or actions) while ignoring others.

Semantic long-term memory (LTM)—the part of declarative or explicit LTM that stores facts about the world, as opposed to distinct episodes.

Semantics—meaning and interpretation of words, phrases, and sentences.

Sensory memory—the very brief retention (for milliseconds to seconds) of just-presented sensory information. *See also* Echoic memory and Iconic memory.

Short-term memory (STM)—the retention of information over seconds to minutes, often involving covert rehearsal, to aid completion of a cognitive task. STM is related to *working memory* and contrasts with *sensory memory* and *long-term memory (LTM)*.

Simultagnosia—inability of an individual to perceive more than a single object at a time, simultagnosia is a defining symptom of *Bálint syndrome*.

Stereopsis—ability to see the external world in three dimensions, even though the input to each retina is two-dimensional.

Substance dualism—in philosophy, the view that the universe contains two fundamental types of entity or substance, mental and physical. Substance dualism is a view of the mind–body problem that was espoused by Plato and Descartes. The contrasting view is monism, which holds there is only one kind of substance in the universe, either matter (*see* Materialism) or mind (*idealism*). In contemporary work on the philosophy of mind, the main contending positions are various forms of materialism or weaker forms of dualism (e.g., property dualism), whereas idealism is mainly of historical interest. *See also* Mind–body problem.

Substantia nigra (SN)—a cluster of nuclei in the midbrain that release dopamine mainly to the basal ganglia to regulate behavior. Dopamine plays an important role in reward learning, addiction, attention, and movement.

Subtraction model—a model of brain function/dysfunction that assumes that a loss of one brain–behavior component does not affect the functions of the remaining brain–behavior components. *See also* Pure insertion.

Sustained attention—a form of attention in which selective attention is maintained over several minutes or longer. *See also* Selective attention; Vigilance.

Synesthesia—adding an extrasensory dimension to a stimulus, such as seeing a black-and-white letter in color.

Syntax—a level of language processing concerned with the relations among the concepts denoted by single words (called grammar in popular usage), syntactic relations are coded mainly by word order, but also by endings attached to single words (like -*s* for plurals and -*ed* for past tense).

Transcortical mixed aphasia—a subtype of aphasia caused by damage around but not in the left hemisphere perisylvian language areas, resulting in impairments in speech fluency (similar to Broca's aphasia) and comprehension (similar to Wernicke's aphasia), but repetition is spared. These patients often have echolalia. Also called isolation of the speech areas. *See other aphasia subtypes.*

Transcortical motor aphasia—a subtype of aphasia caused by damage in the left frontal lobe outside Broca's area in which speech fluency is impaired and comprehension is intact (like Broca's aphasia), but repetition is spared. These patients often have echolalia. *See other aphasia subtypes.*

Transcortical sensory aphasia—a subtype of aphasia caused by damage in the posterior left hemisphere outside Wernicke's area in which comprehension is impaired and fluency is intact (like Wernicke's aphasia), but repetition is intact with echolalia. *See other aphasia subtypes.*

Transparency assumption—transparency assumes a simple one-to-one correspondence between components of behavior and components of brain. This assumption is required for the subtraction model to be valid.

Ventral syndrome—one of three neurological syndromes caused by damage to the prefrontal cortex (PFC), the ventral syndrome is caused by damage to the orbitofrontal or ventromedial PFC and produces what is called pseudopsychopathic behavior, marked by socially inappropriate comments and actions. These behaviors include sexually inappropriate behavior and incontinence. *See also* Lateral syndrome; Medial syndromes.

Ventral tegmental area (VTA)—a collection of neurons in the midbrain that releases dopamine into the prefrontal cortex and limbic areas to regulate behavior. *See also* Substantia nigra (SN).

Ventral visual pathway—the visual pathway from the occipital lobe into the temporal cortex that is specialized for identifying visual objects. *See also* Dorsal visual pathway.

Vestibular ocular reflex—a compensatory eye movement that stabilizes images on the retina during head movement, this reflex is an example of *corollary discharge*.

Vigilance—another name for *sustained attention*.

Wernicke's aphasia—a subtype of aphasia caused by damage to Wernicke's area in the left posterior hemisphere, in which comprehension and repetition of language is impaired, but fluency is preserved. *See other aphasia subtypes.*

Word superiority effect—a seemingly paradoxical experimental phenomenon in which recognition of a letter presented within words or pseudowords is superior to recognition of a letter presented by itself. *See also* Interactive activation model.

Working memory—a subtype of transient memory that requires concurrent storage and processing of information. *See also* Short-term memory (STM).

References

Adolphs, R. (2003). Cognitive neuroscience of human social behaviour. *Nature Reviews Neuroscience, 4*(3), 165–178.

Agin, D. (2010). *More than genes.* New York: Oxford University Press.

Albin, R. L., & Mink, J. W. (2006). Recent advances in Tourette syndrome research. *Trends in Neuroscience, 29*(3), 175–182.

Alloy, L. B., Abramson, L. Y., Walshaw, P. D., Cogswell, A., Grandin, L. D., Hughes, M. E., et al. (2008). Behavioral approach system and behavioral inhibition system sensitivities and bipolar spectrum disorders: Prospective prediction of bipolar mood episodes. *Bipolar Disorders, 10*(2), 310–322.

Anderson, J. R. (1983). *The architecture of cognition.* Cambridge, MA: MIT Press.

Atkinson, R. C., & Shiffrin, R. M. (1968). Human memory: A proposed system and its control processes. In K. W. Spence & J. T. Spence (Eds.), *The psychology of learning and motivation* (Vol. 2, pp. 89–195). New York: Academic Press.

Avidan, G., & Behrmann, M. (2008). Implicit familiarity processing in congenital prosopagnosia. *Journal of Neuropsychology, 2*(Pt. 1), 141–164.

Baars, B. (1989). *A cognitive theory of consciousness.* Cambridge, MA: Cambridge University Press.

Baars, B. J., & Gage, N. M. (2010). *Cognition, brain, and consciousness.* New York: Elsevier.

Bachevalier, J., & Mishkin, M. (1984). An early and a late developing system for learning and retention in infant monkeys. *Behavioral Neuroscience, 98*(5), 770–778.

Banich, M. T., & Compton, R. J. (2011). *Cognitive neuroscience* (3rd ed.). Belmont, CA: Wadsworth, Cengage Learning.

Barnes, K. A., Howard, J. H., Jr., Howard, D. V., Kenealy, L., & Vaidya, C. J. (2010). Two forms of implicit learning in childhood ADHD. *Developmental Neuropsychology, 35*(5), 494–505.

Barrett, L. F. (2012). Emotions are real. *Emotion, 12*(3), 413–429.

Bartlett, F. C. (1932). *Remembering: A study in experimental and social psychology.* Cambridge, UK: Cambridge University Press.

Bates, E. A. (1998). Construction grammar and its implications for child language research. *Journal of Child Language, 25,* 462–466.

Bates, E. A. (2004). Explaining and interpreting deficits in language development across clinical groups: Where do we go from here? *Brain and Language, 88*(2), 248–253.

Bates, E. A., & Goodman, J. C. (1997). On the inseparability of grammar and the lexicon: Evidence from acquisition, aphasia and real-time processing. *Language and Cognitive Processes, 12*(5/6), 507–584.

Bates, E. A., & MacWhinney, B. (1988). "What is functionalism?" *Papers and Reports on Child Language Development, 27,* 137–152.

Bates, E. A., & Roe, K. (2001). Language development in children with unilateral brain injury. In C. A. Nelson & M. Luciana (Eds.), *Handbook of developmental cognitive neuroscience* (pp. 281–307). Cambridge, MA: MIT Press.

Bechara, A., Tranel, D., Damasio, H., Adolfs, R., Rockland, C., & Damasio, A. R. (1995). Double dissociation of conditioning and declarative knowledge relative to the amygdala and hippocampus in humans. *Science, 269,* 1115–1118.

Bellugi, U., Marks, S., Bihrle, A., & Sabo, H. (1988). Dissociations between language and cognitive functions in Williams syndrome. In D. V. M. Bishop & K. Mogford (Eds.), *Language development in exceptional circumstances* (pp. 177–189). Edinburgh, Scotland: Churchill Livingstone.

Benes, F. M. (1993). Neurobiological investigations in cingulate cortex of schizophrenic brain. *Schizophrenia Bulletin, 19*(3), 537–549.

Berger, H. (1929). Über des elektrenkephalogramm des menchen. *Archives für Psychiatrie und Nervenkrankheiten, 87,* 527–580.

Bergson, H. (1907). *Creative evolution* (A. Mitchell, Trans.). New York: Modern Library, 1911.

Berk, L. E. (2005). *Infants and children* (5th ed.). New York: Pearson Education.

Bernat, J. L. (2009). Chronic consciousness disorders. *Annual Review of Medicine, 60,* 381–392.

Berridge, C. W., & Devilbiss, D. M. (2011). Psychostimulants as cognitive enhancers: The prefrontal cortex, catecholamines, and attention-deficit/hyperactivity disorder. *Biological Psychiatry, 69*(12), e101–e111.

Berridge, K. C. (2003). Pleasures of the brain. *Brain and Cognition, 52*(1), 106–128.

Berridge, K. C. (2009). "Liking" and "wanting" food rewards: Brain substrates and roles in eating disorders. *Physiological Behavior, 97*(5), 537–550.

Best, C. T., McRoberts, G. W., & Goodell, E. (2001). Discrimination of non-native consonant contrasts varying in perceptual assimilation to the listener's native phonological system. *Journal of the Acoustic Society of America, 109,* 775–794.

Bhatt, R. S., Bertin, E., Hayden, A., & Reed, A. (2005). Face processing in infancy: Developmental changes in the use of different kinds of relational information. *Child Development, 76*(1), 169–181.

Bird, C. M., & Burgess, N. (2008). The hippocampus and memory: Insights from spatial processing. *Nature Reviews Neuroscience, 9,* 182–194.

Bird, J., & Bishop, D. V. M. (1992). Perception and awareness of phonemes in phonologically impaired children. *European Journal of Disorders of Communication, 27*(4), 289–311.

Bishop, D. V. M. (1985). Spelling ability in congenital dysarthria: Evidence against articulatory coding in translating between phonemes and graphemes. *Cognitive Neuropsychology, 2*(3), 229–251.

Bishop, D. V. M. (1997). *Uncommon understanding: Development and disorders of language comprehension in children*. Hove, East Sussex, UK: Psychology Press.

Bishop, D. V. M. (2006). Developmental cognitive genetics: How psychology can inform genetics and vice versa. *Quarterly Journal of Experimental Psychology, 59*, 1153–1168.

Bishop, D. V. M., Bishop, S. J., Bright, P., James, C., Delaney, T., & Tallal, P. (1999). Different origin of auditory and phonological processing problems in children with language impairment: Evidence from a twin study. *Journal of Speech, Language and Hearing Research, 42*(1), 155–168.

Bishop, D. V. M., McDonald, D., & Bird, S. (2009). Why do language and literacy problems co-occur in children? Evaluation of a multiple overlapping risk factors (mcrf) model.

Bishop, D. V. M., McDonald, D., Bird, S., & Hayiou-Thomas, M. E. (2009). Children who read words accurately despite language impairment: Who are they and how do they do it? *Child Development, 80*(2), 593–605.

Bishop, D. V. M., & Snowling, M. J. (2004). Developmental dyslexia and specific language impairment: Same or different? *Psychological Bulletin, 130*(6), 858–886.

Bisiach, E., Geminiani, G., Berti, A., & Rusconi, M. L. (1990). Perceptual and premotor factors of unilateral neglect. *Neurology, 40*(8), 1278–1281.

Bisiach, E., & Luzzatti, C. (1978). Unilateral neglect of representational space. *Cortex, 14*(1), 129–133.

Bisiach, E., Neppi-Modona, M., & Ricci, R. (2002). Space anisometry in unilateral neglect. In H. O. Karnath, A. D. Milner, & G. Villar (Eds.), *The cognitive and neural bases of spatial neglect* (pp. 145–152). Oxford, UK: Oxford University Press.

Blakemore, S. J., & Frith, C. D. (2003). Disorders of self-monitoring and the symptoms of schizophrenia. In T. Kircher & A. David (Eds.), *The self in neuroscience and psychiatry* (pp. 407–424). New York: Cambridge University Press.

Bliss, T. V., & Lømo, T. (1973). Long-lasting potentiation of synaptic transmission in the dentate area of the anaesthetized rabbit following stimulation of the perforant path. *Journal of Physiology, 232*(2), 331–356.

Boada, R., & Pennington, B. F. (2006). Deficient implicit phonological representations in children with dyslexia. *Journal of Experimental Child Psychology, 95*(3), 153–193.

Boller, F., & Duyckaerts, C. (2003). Alzheimer's disease: Clinical and anatomic issues. In T. E. Feinberg & M. J. Farah (Eds.), *Behavioral neurology and neuropsychology* (pp. 515–543). New York: McGraw-Hill.

Botvinick, M., & Cohen, J. (1998). Rubber hands "feel" touch that eyes see. *Nature, 391*(6669), 756.

Broca, P. (1861). Nouvelle observation d'aphémie produite par une lésion de la moitié postérieure des deuxième et troisième circonvolutions frontales gauches. *Bulletin of the Society of Anatomy, 36*, 398–407.

Broomfield, J., & Dodd, B. (2001). Mainstream paediatric speech and language therapy service population: Epidemiology. *International Journal of Language and Communication Disorders, 36Suppl*, 447–452.

Brown, J. (1972). *Aphasia, apraxia and agnosia*. Springfield, IL: Charles C. Thomas.

Brown, R. (1973). *The first language*. Cambridge, MA: Harvard University Press.

Bryson, C. Q. (1970). Systematic identification of perceptual disabilities in autistic children. *Perception and Motor Skills, 31*(1), 239–246.

Buckner, R. L. (2010). The role of the hippocampus in prediction and imagination. *Annual Reviews in Psychology, 61*, 27–48, C21–C28.

Burdach, K. F. (1819). Personality changes after operations of the frontal lobes. *Acta Psychiatrica et Neurologica Scandanavia, 20.*

Byrne, B., & Shea, P. (1979). Semantic and phonetic memory codes in beginning readers. *Memory and Cognition, 7*(5), 333–338.

Cain, K., Oakhill, J., & Lemmon, K. (2004). Individual differences in the inference of word meanings from context. *Journal of Educational Psychology, 96*, 671–681.

Campbell, R., Pascalis, O., Coleman, M., Wallace, B., & Benson, P. J. (1997). Are faces of different species perceived categorically by human observers? *Proceedings of the Royal Society B: London of Biological Sciences, 264*, 1429–1434.

Campbell, T. F., Dollaghan, C. A., Rockette, H. E., Paradise, J. L., Feldman, H. M., Shriberg, L. D., et al. (2003). Risk factors for speech delay of unknown origin in 3-year-old children. *Child Development, 74*(2), 346–357.

Caplan, D. (2003). Aphasic syndromes. In K. M. Heilman & E. Valenstein (Eds.), *Clinical neuropsychology* (4th ed., pp. 14–34). New York: Oxford University Press.

Card, J. P., Swanson, L. W., & Moore, R. Y. (2008). The hypothalamus: An overview of regulatory systems. In L. R. Squire, D. Berg, F. E. Bloom, S. du Lac, A. Ghosh, & N. C. Spitzer (Eds.), *Fundamental neruroscience* (3rd ed., pp. 795–806). New York: Elsevier.

Carey, S., & Diamond, R. (1977). From piecemeal to configurational representation of faces. *Science, 195*(4275), 312–314.

Carpenter, P. A., Just, M. A., & Shell, P. (1990). What one intelligence test measures: A theoretical account of the processing in the raven progressive matrices test. *Psychological Review, 97*(3), 404–431.

Castles, A., & Coltheart, M. (2004). Is there a causal link from phonological awareness to success in learning to read? *Cognition, 91*, 77–111.

Cavanagh, J. F., Bismark, A. J., Frank, M. J., & Allen, J. J. (2011). Larger error signals in major depression are associated with better avoidance learning. *Frontiers in Psychology, 2*, 331.

Chalmers, D. J. (1998). The problems of consciousness. *Advances in Neurology, 77*, 7–16.

Chase, H. W., Frank, M. J., Michael, A., Bullmore, E. T., Sahakian, B. J., & Robbins, T. W. (2010). Approach and avoidance learning in patients with major depression and healthy controls: Relation to anhedonia. *Psychological Medicine, 40*(3), 433–440.

Choi, J. S., Kang, D. H., Kim, J. J., Ha, T. H., Roh, K. S., Youn, T., et al. (2005). Decreased caudal anterior cingulate gyrus volume and positive symptoms in schizophrenia. *Psychiatry Research, 139*(3), 239–247.

Chomsky, N. (1959). Review of Skinner's verbal behavior. *Language, 35*, 26–58.

Churchland, P. (2013). *Touching a nerve.* New York: Norton.

Churchland, P. M. (1995). *The engine of reason, the seat of the soul.* Cambridge, MA: MIT Press.

Churchland, P. S. (1986). *Neurophilosophy: Toward a unified science of the mind–brain.* Cambridge, MA: MIT Press.

Coltheart, M. (1989). From neuropsychology to mental structure. *Science, 246*(4931), 827–828.

Colvin, A. N., Yeates, K. O., Enrile, B. G., & Coury, D. L. (2003). Motor adaptation in children with myelomeningocele: Comparison to children with ADHD and healthy siblings. *Journal of the International Neuropsychological Society, 9*(4), 642–652.

Corriveau, K., Pasquini, E., & Goswami, U. (2007). Basic auditory processing skills and specific language impairment: A new look at an old hypothesis. *Journal of Speech, Language and Hearing Research, 50*(3), 647–666.

Costa, V. D., Lang, P. J., Sabatinelli, D., Versace, F., & Bradley, M. M. (2010). Emotional imagery: Assessing pleasure and arousal in the brain's reward circuitry. *Human Brain Mapping, 31*(9), 1446–1457.

Cowey, A., & Heywood, C. A. (1997). Cerebral achromatopsia: Colour blindness despite wavelength processing. *Trends in Cognitive Sciences, 1*(4), 133–139.

Crone, E. A., & Westenberg, P. M. (2009). A brain-based account of developmental changes. In M. de Haan & M. R. Gunnar (Eds.), *Handbook of developmental social neuroscience* (pp. 378–398). New York: Guilford Press.

Curtis, M. E. (1980). Development of components of reading skill. *Journal of Educational Psychology, 72*, 656–669.

Damasio, A. R. (1994). *Descartes' error: Emotion, reason, and the human brain.* New York: G. P. Putnam's Sons.

Damasio, A. R. (2010). *Self comes to mind: Constructing the conscious brain.* New York: Pantheon Books.

D'Angiulli, A., & Siegel, L. S. (2003). Cognitive functioning as measured by the WISC-R: Do children with learning disabilities have distinctive patterns of performance? *Journal of Learning Disabilities, 36*(1), 48–58.

Dawkins, R. (1987). *The blind watchmaker: Why the evidence of evolution reveals a universe without design.* New York: Norton.

DeGutis, J., & D'Esposito, M. (2007). Distinct mechanisms in visual category learning. *Cognitive Affective Behavioral Neuroscience, 7*(3), 251–259.

de Haan, M., Mishkin, M., Baldeweg, T., & Vargha-Khadem, F. (2006). Human memory development and its dysfunction after early hippocampal injury. *Trends in Neurosciences, 29*(7), 374–381.

Dennett, D. C. (1987). *The intentional stance.* Cambridge, MA: MIT Press.

Depue, R. A., & Iacono, W. G. (1989). Neurobehavioral aspects of affective disorders. *Annual Review of Psychology, 40*, 457–492.

Desimone, R., & Duncan, J. (1995). Neural mechanisms of selective visual attention. *Annual Review of Neuroscience, 18*, 193–222.

Diamond, A. (1989). Developmental progression in human infants and infant monkeys, and the neural bases of inhibitory control of reaching. In *The development and neural bases of higher cognitive functions* (pp. 637–639). New York: Academy of Science Press.

Diamond, A., & Goldman-Rakic, P. S. (1989). Comparison of human infants and infant rhesus monkeys on Piaget's AB task: Evidence for dependence on dorsolateral prefrontal cortex. *Experimental Brain Research, 74*, 24–40.

Diamond, A., Werker, J. F., & Lalonde, C. (1994). Toward understanding common-alities in the development of object search, detour navigation, categorization and speech perception. In G. Dawson & K. W. Fisher (Eds.), *Human behavior and the developing brain* (pp. 380–426). New York: Guilford Press.

Dobzhansky, T. (1973). Nothing in biology makes sense except in the light of evolu-tion. *American Biology Teacher, 35*(3), 125–129.

Donald, M. (2001). *A mind so rare.* New York: Norton.

Drevets, W. C., Price, J. L., & Furey, M. L. (2008). Brain structural and functional abnormalities in mood disorders: Implications for neurocircuitry models of depression. *Brain Structure and Function, 213*(1–2), 93–118.

Driver, J., Baylis, G. C., & Rafal, R. D. (1993). Preserved figure-ground segregation and symmetry perception in a patient with neglect. *Nature, 360*(6399), 73–75.

Drummey, A. B., & Newcombe, N. (1995). Remembering versus knowing the past: Children's explicit and implicit memories for pictures. *Journal of Experimental Child Psychology, 59*(3), 549–565.

Duchaine, B. C., & Nakayama, K. (2006). Developmental prosopagnosia: A win-dow to content-specific face processing. *Current Opinions in Neurobiology, 16*(2), 166–173.

Duncan, J. (2001). An adaptive coding model of neural function in prefrontal cortex. *Nature Reviews Neuroscience, 2,* 820–829.

Duncan, J., Burgess, P., & Emslie, H. (1995). Fluid intelligence after frontal lobe lesions. *Neuropsychologia, 33*(3), 261–268.

Dunn, J. C., & Kirsner, K. (1988). Discovering functionally independent mental pro-cesses: The principle of reversed association. *Psychological Review, 95*(1), 91–101.

Durrell, L. (1962). *The Alexandria quartet.* London, Faber: Faber.

Edgin, J. O., Pennington, B. F., & Mervis, C. B. (2010). Neuropsychological com-ponents of intellectual disability: The contributions of immediate, working, and associative memory. *Journal of Intellectual Disability Research, 54*(5), 406–417.

Eglin, M., Robertson, L. C., & Knight, R. T. (1989). Visual search performance in the neglect syndrome. *Journal of Cognitive Neuroscience, 1,* 372–385.

Eimer, M., Gosling, A., & Duchaine, B. (2012). Electrophysiological markers of covert face recognition in developmental prosopagnosia. *Brain, 135*(Pt. 2), 542–554.

Ekman, P. (2003). *Emotions revealed.* New York: Times Books.

Elbro, C., Borstrom, I., & Petersen, D. (1998). Predicting dyslexia from kindergar-ten: The importance of distinctness of phonological representations of lexical items. *Reading Research Quarterly, 33,* 36–60.

Ellis, A. W. (1987). Intimations of modularity, or the modularity of mind: Doing cognitive neuropsychology without syndromes. In M. Coltheart, G. Sartori, & R. Job (Eds.), *The cognitive neuropsychology of language* (pp. 397–408). London: Erlbaum.

Elman, J. L., Bates, E. A., Johnson, M. H., Karmiloff-Smith, A., Parisi, D., & Plun-kett, K. (1996). *Rethinking innateness: Connectionist perspectives on development.* Cambridge, MA: MIT Press.

Etkin, A., & Wager, T. D. (2007). Functional neuroimaging of anxiety: A meta-analysis of emotional processing in PTSD, social anxiety disorder, and specific phobia. *American Journal of Psychiatry, 164*(10), 1476–1488.

Etkin, A., & Wager, T. D. (2010). Brain systems underlying anxiety disorders: A view from neuroimaging. In H. B. Simpson, F. Schneier, Y. Neria, & R. Lewis-Fernandez (Eds.), *Anxiety disorders: Theory, research and clinical perspectives* (pp. 192–203). Cambridge, UK: Cambridge University Press.

Farah, M. J. (1994). Neuropsychological inference with an interactive brain. *Behavioral and Brain Sciences, 17*, 90–104.

Farah, M. J. (2003). Computational modeling in behavioral neurology and neuropsychology. In T. E. Feinberg & J. J. Farah (Eds.), *Behavioral neurology and neuropsychology* (pp. 135–143). New York: McGraw-Hill.

Ferrier, D. (1886). *The function of the brain.* London: Smith, Elder.

Ferro, J. M., Martins, I. P., & Tavora, L. (1984). Neglect in children. *Annals of Neurology, 15*(3), 281–284.

Filley, C. M. (2011). *Neurobehavioral anatomy* (3rd ed.). Boulder, CO: University Press of Colorado.

Finger, S. (1994). *Origins of neuroscience.* New York: Oxford University Press.

Fletcher, J. M., Foorman, B. R., Shaywitz, S. E., Shaywitz, B. A., & Tager-Flusberg, H. (1999). Conceptual and methodological issues in dyslexia research: A lesson for developmental disorders. In *Neurodevelopmental disorders* (pp. 271–305). Cambridge, MA: MIT Press.

Flor, H., Elbert, T., Knecht, S., Wienbruch, C., Pantev, C., Birbaumer, N., et al. (1995). Phantom-limb pain as a perceptual correlate of cortical reorganization following arm amputation. *Nature, 375*, 482–484.

Fodor, J. A. (1983). *The modularity of mind.* Cambridge, MA: MIT Press.

Fowler, A. E. (1991). How early phonological development might set the stage for phoneme awareness. In S. A. Brady & D. P. Shankweiler (Eds.), *Phonological processes in literacy: A tribute to Isabelle Y. Liberman* (pp. 97–117). Hillsdale, NJ: Erlbaum.

Fowler, A. E., & Swainson, B. (2004). Relationships of naming skills to reading, memory, and receptive vocabulary: Evidence for imprecise phonological representations of words by poor readers. *Annals of Dyslexia, 54*(2), 247–280.

Fox, M. D., Snyder, A. Z., Vincent, J. L., Corbetta, M., Van Essen, D. C., & Raichle, M. E. (2005). The human brain is intrinsically organized into dynamic, anticorrelated functional networks. *Proceedings of the National Academy of Sciences USA, 102*, 9673–9678.

Frank, M. J., Santamaria, A., O'Reilly, R. C., & Willcutt, E. (2007). Testing computational models of dopamine and noradrenaline dysfunction in attention deficit/hyperactivity disorder. *Neuropsychopharmacology, 32*(7), 1583–1599.

Frank, M. J., Seeberger, L. C., & O'Reilly R, C. (2004). By carrot or by stick: Cognitive reinforcement learning in parkinsonism. *Science, 306*(5703), 1940–1943.

Freedman, D. J., Riesenhuber, M., Poggio, T., & Miller, E. K. (2001). Categorical representation of visual stimuli in the primate prefrontal cortex. *Science, 291*(5502), 312–316.

Freud, S. (1953). *On aphasia: A critical study* (E. Stengel, Trans.). New York: International Universities Press. (Original work published 1891)

Friederici, A. D., von Cramon, D. Y., & Kotz, S. A. (2007). Role of the corpus callosum in speech comprehension: Interfacing syntax and prosody. *Neuron, 53*(1), 135–145.

Frith, C. D. (1987). The positive and negative symptoms of schizophrenia reflect impairments in the perception and initiation of action. *Psychological Medicine, 17*(3), 631–648.

Frith, C. D., & Done, D. J. (1989). Experiences of alien control in schizophrenia reflect a disorder in the central monitoring of action. *Psychological Medicine, 19*(2), 359–363.

Fritsch, G., & Hitzig, E. (1870). On the electrical excitability of the cerebrum (G. Von Bonin, Trans.). In *Some papers on the cerebral cortex* (pp. 73–96). Springfield, IL: Charles C. Thomas.

Fuster, J. M. (1989). *The prefrontal cortex: Anatomy, physiology and neuropsychology of the frontal lobe* (2nd ed.). New York: Raven.

Gall, F. J., & Spurzheim, G. (1809). Research on the nervous system in general and on that of the brain in particular. In K. Pribram (Ed.), *Brain and behaviour: Mood states and mind* (Vol. 1, pp. 20–27). Harmondsworth, UK: Penguin Books.

Garber, K. B., Visootsak, J., & Warren, S. T. (2008). Fragile X syndrome. *European Journal of Human Genetics, 16*(6), 666–672.

Gardner, H. (1983). *Frames of mind.* New York: Basic Books.

Gathercole, S. E., & Baddeley, A. D. (1990a). Phonological memory deficits in language disordered children: Is there a causal connection? *Journal of Memory and Language, 29*(3), 336.

Gathercole, S. E., & Baddeley, A. D. (1990b). The role of phonological memory in vocabulary acquisition: A study of young children learning new names. *British Journal of Developmental Psychology, 81*, 439–454.

Gauthier, I., & Nelson, C. (2001). The development of face expertise. *Current Opinion in Neurobiology, 11*, 219–224.

Gauthier, I., Skudlarski, P., Gore, J. C., & Anderson, A. W. (2000). Expertise for cars and birds recruits brain areas involved in face recognition. *Nature Neuroscience, 3*(2), 191–197.

Gauthier, I., Tarr, M. J., Anderson, A. W., Skudlarski, P., & Gore, J. C. (1999). Activation of the middle fusiform "face area" increases with expertise in recognizing novel objects. *Nature Neuroscience, 2*(6), 568–573.

Gazzaniga, M. S., Ivry, R. B., & Magnun, G. R. (2009). *Cognitive neuroscience: The biology of the mind* (3rd ed.). New York: Norton.

Gibbs, F. A., & Gibbs, E. L. (1948). Psychiatric implications of discharging temporal lobe lesions. *Translation of the American Neurology Association, 73*, 133–137.

Gillihan, S. J., & Farah, M. J. (2005). Is self special? A critical review of evidence from experimental psychology and cognitive neuroscience. *Psychological Bulletin, 131*(1), 76–97.

Gödel, K. (1931). Die kvollständigkeit der axiome des logischen funktionenkalküls. *Monatshefte für Mathematik und Physik, 37*, 349–360.

Golarai, G., Ghahremani, D. G., Whitfield-Gabrieli, S., Reiss, A., Eberhardt, J. L., Gabrieli, J. D., et al. (2007). Differential development of high-level visual cortex correlates with category-specific recognition memory. *National Neuroscience, 10*(4), 512–522.

Goldman-Rakic, P. S. (1987). Development of cortical circuitry and cognitive function. *Child Development, 58*(3), 601–622.

Goldman-Rakic, P. S. (1993). Working memory and the mind. In *Mind and brain* (pp. 67–77). New York: Freeman.

Goldsmith, T. H. (1991). *The biological roots of human nature*. New York: Oxford University Press.

Goldstein, K. (1948). *Language and language disturbance*. New York: Grune & Stratton.

Goltz, F. (1888).Über die verrichtungen des grosshirns. *Archives of Gestational Physiology, 42*, 419–467.

Gopnik, M., & Crago, M. B. (1991). Familial aggregation of a developmental language disorder. *Cognition, 39*(1), 1–50.

Goswami, U., Thomson, J., Richardson, U., Stainthorp, R., Hughes, D., Rosen, S., et al. (2002). Amplitude envelope onsets and developmental dyslexia: A new hypothesis. *Proceedings of the National Academy of Sciences USA, 99*(16), 10911–10916.

Gotlib, I. H., & Hamilton, J. P. (2008). Neuroimaging and depression. *Current Directions in Psychological Science, 17*(2), 159–163.

Graf Estes, K., Evans, J. L., & Else-Quest, N. M. (2007). Differences in the nonword repetition performance of children with and without specific language impairment: A meta-analysis. *Journal of Speech, Language, and Hearing Research, 50*(1), 177–195.

Grafman, J. (2002). The human prefrontal cortex has evolved to represent components of structured event compensation. In *Handbook of neuropsychology* (pp. 157–174). Amsterdam: Elsevier.

Gray, J. A. (1982). *The neuropsychology of anxiety*. Oxford, UK: Oxford University Press.

Greenough, W. T., Black, J. E., & Wallace, C. S. (1987). Experience and brain development. *Child Development, 58*(3), 539–559.

Gregory, R. L. (1961). The brain as an engineering problem. In W. H. Thorpe & O. L. Zangwill (Eds.), *Current problems in animal behavior* (pp. 307–330). Cambridge, UK: Cambridge University Press.

Gregory, R. L. (1968). Models and the localization of functions in the central nervous system. In C. R. Evans & A. D. J. Robertson (Eds.), *Key papers in cybernetics* (pp. 91–102). London: Butterworth.

Greicius, M. D., Flores, B. H., Menon, V., Glover, G. H., Solvason, H. B., Kenna, H., et al. (2007). Resting-state functional connectivity in major depression: Abnormally increased contributions from subgenual cingulate cortex and thalamus. *Biological Psychiatry, 62*(5), 429–437.

Grill-Spector, K., Sayres, R., & Ress, D. (2006). High-resolution imaging reveals highly selective nonface clusters in the fusiform face area. *Nature Neuroscience, 9*(9), 1177–1185.

Guenther, F. H. (1995). Speech sound acquisition, coarticulation, and rate effects in a neural network model of speech production. *Psychology Review, 102*(3), 594–621.

Gusnard, D. A., & Raichle, M. E. (2001). Searching for a baseline: Functional imaging and the resting human brain. *Nature Reviews Neuroscience, 2*(10), 685–694.

Haith, M. M. (1966). The response of the human newborn to visual movement. *Journal of Experimental Child Psychology, 3*, 235–243.

Haith, M. M., Benson, J. B., Roberts, R. J., Jr., & Pennington, B. F. (1994). *The development of future-oriented processes*. Chicago: University of Chicago Press.

Haith, M. M., Hazan, C., & Goodman, G. S. (1988). Expectation and anticipation of dynamic visual events by 3.5-month-old babies. *Child Development, 59*(2), 467–479.

Hamilton, J. P., Chen, G., Thomason, M. E., Schwartz, M. E., & Gotlib, I. H. (2012). Investigating neural primacy in major depressive disorder: Multivariate Granger causality analysis of resting-state fMRI time-series data. *Molecular Psychiatry, 16*(7), 763–772.

Hanson, S. J., & Halchenko, Y. O. (2008). Brain reading using full brain support vector machines for object recognition: There is no "face" identification area. *Neural Computation, 20,* 486–503.

Hardy, J., & Selkoe, D. J. (2002). The amyloid hypothesis of Alzheimer's disease: Progress and problems on the road to therapeutics. *Science, 297*(5580), 353–356.

Harlow, J. M. (1993). Recovery from the passage of an iron bar through the head. *History of Psychiatry, 4*(14), 274–281. (Original work published 1868)

Harm, M. W., & Seidenberg, M. S. (1999). Phonology, reading acquisition, and dyslexia: Insights from connectionist models. *Psychological Review, 106*(3), 491–528.

Harm, M. W., & Seidenberg, M. S. (2004). Computing the meanings of words in reading: Cooperative division of labor between visual and phonological processes. *Psychological Review, 111*(3), 662–720.

Hassabis, D., Kumaran, D., Vann, S. D., & Maguire, E. A. (2007). Patients with hippocampal amnesia cannot imagine new experiences. *Proceedings of the National Academy of Sciences USA, 104*(5), 1726–1731.

Haxby, J. V., Gobbini, M. I., Furey, M. L., Ishai, A., Schouten, J. L., & Pietrini, P. (2001). Distributed and overlapping representations of faces and objects in ventral temporal cortex. *Science, 293*(5539), 2425–2430.

Hayne, H. (2004). Infant memory development: Implications for childhood amnesia. *Developmental Review, 24,* 33–73.

Head, H. (1926). *Aphasia and kindred disorders of speech.* Cambridge, UK: Cambridge University Press.

Hebb, D. O. (1945). Man's frontal lobes: A critical review. *Archives of Neurological Psychiatry, 54,* 10–24.

Hebb, D. O. (1949). *The organization of behavior.* New York: Wiley.

Heilman, K. M., Maher, L. M., Greenwald, M. L., & Rothi, L. J. (1997). Conceptual apraxia from lateralized lesions. *Neurology, 49*(2), 457–464.

Heilman, K. M., & Valenstein, E. (2003). *Clinical neuropsychology.* New York: Oxford University Press.

Hillis, A. E., Newhart, M., Heidler, J., Barker, P. B., Herskovits, E. H., & Degaonkar, M. (2005). Anatomy of spatial attention: Insights from perfusion imaging and hemispatial neglect in acute stroke. *Journal of Neuroscience, 25*(12), 3161–3167.

Hinton, G. E., & Sejnowski, T. J. (1986). Learning and relearning in Boltzman machines. In D. E. Rumelhart & J. L. McClelland (Eds.), *Parallel distributed processing* (Vol. 1, pp. 282–317). Cambridge, MA: MIT Press.

Hinton, G. E., & Shallice, T. (1991). Lesioning an attractor network: Investigations of acquired dyslexia. *Psychological Review, 98,* 96–121.

Hoeft, F., Carter, J. C., Lightbody, A. A., Cody Hazlett, H., Piven, J., & Reiss, A. L. (2010). Region-specific alterations in brain development in one- to three-year-old boys with fragile X syndrome. *Proceedings of the National Academy of Sciences USA, 107*(20), 9335–9339.

Hofstader, D. (1980). *Gödel, Escher, Bach*. New York: Vintage.

Hoover, W. A., & Gough, P. B. (1990). The simple view of reading. *Reading and Writing: An Interdisciplinary Journal, 2*, 127–160.

Hornik, K., Stinchcombe, M., & White, H. (1989). Multilayer feedforward networks are universal approximator. *Neural Networks, 2*(5), 359–366.

Hubel, D. H., & Wiesel, T. N. (1998). Early exploration of the visual cortex. *Neuron, 20*(3), 401–412.

Hughlings Jackson, J. (1931). *Selected writings of John Hughlings Jackson* (Vols. 1 and 2). London: Hodder.

Ingvar, D. H. (1979). "Hyperfrontal" distribution of the cerebral grey matter flow in resting wakefulness: On the functional anatomy of the conscious state. *Acta Neurologica Scandinavica, 60*, 12–25.

Izard, C. E. (1992). Basic emotions, relations among emotions, and emotion-cognition relations. *Psychological Review, 99*(3), 561–565.

Jakobson, R. (1941). *Child, language, aphasia and phonological universals*. The Hague: Mouton Publishers.

James, W. (1890). *The principles of psychology* (Vol. 1). New York: Holt.

Jeannerod, M., Farrer, C., Franck, N., Fourneret, P., Posada, A., Daprati, E., et al. (2003). Action recognition in normal and schizophrenic subjects. In T. Kircher & A. David (Eds.), *The self in neuroscience and psychiatry* (pp. 380–406). New York: Cambridge University Press.

Joanisse, M. F. (2000). *Connectionist phonology*. Unpublished PhD dissertation. University of Southern California.

Joanisse, M. F. (2004). Specific language impairments in children: Phonology, semantics, and the English past tense. *Current Directions in Psychological Science, 13*(4), 156.

Joanisse, M. F. (2007). Phonological deficits and developmental language impairments: Evidence from connectionist models. In D. Mareschal, S. Sirois, G. Westermann, & M. H. Johnson (Eds.), *Neuroconstructionism: Perspectives and prospects* (Vol. 2, pp. 205–229). Oxford, UK: Oxford University Press.

Joanisse, M. F., & Seidenberg, M. S. (2003). Phonology and syntax in specific language impairment: Evidence from a connectionist model. *Brain and Language, 86*(1), 40.

Johnson, E. P., Pennington, B. F., Lowenstein, J. H., & Nittrouer, S. (2011). Sensitivity to structure in the speech signal by children with speech sound disorder and reading disability. *Journal of Communication Disorders, 44*, 294–314.

Johnson, M. H. (1990). *The body in the mind*. Chicago: University of Chicago Press.

Johnson, M. H., & de Haan, M. (2011). *Developmental cognitive neuroscience*. Oxford, UK: Blackwell.

Johnston, R. S. (1982). Phonological coding in dyslexic readers. *British Journal of Psychology, 73*, 455–460.

Kandel, E. R., & Hawkins, R. D. (1993). The biological basis of learning and individuality. In *Readings from Scientific American* (pp. 40–53). New York: Freeman.

Kanwisher, N. (2010). Functional specificity in the human brain: A window into the functional architecture of the mind. *Proceedings of the National Academy of Sciences USA, 107*(25), 11163–11170.

Karnath, H. O., Fruhmann Berger, M., Kuker, W., & Rorden, C. (2004). The anatomy of spatial neglect based on voxelwise statistical analysis: A study of 140 patients. *Cerebral Cortex, 14*(10), 1164–1172.

Kenney, M. K., Barac-Cikoja, D., Finnegan, K., Jeffries, N., & Ludlow, C. L. (2006). Speech perception and short-term memory deficits in persistent developmental speech disorder. *Brain and Language, 96*(2), 178–190.

Kerns, J. G., Cohen, J. D., MacDonald, A. W., 3rd, Johnson, M. K., Stenger, V. A., Aizenstein, H., et al. (2005). Decreased conflict- and error-related activity in the anterior cingulate cortex in subjects with schizophrenia. *American Journal of Psychiatry, 162*(10), 1833–1839.

Kimberg, D. Y., D'Esposito, M. D., & Farha, M. J. (1997). Frontal lobes: Cognitive neuropsychological aspects. In T. E. Feinberg & M. J. Farah (Eds.), *Behavioral neurology and neuropsychology* (pp. 409–418). New York: McGraw-Hill.

Kintsch, W. (1994). The psychology of discourse processing. In A. M. Gernsbacher (Ed.), *Handbook of psycholinguistics* (pp. 721–740). San Diego, CA: Academic Press.

Koch, C. (2009, September/October). When does consciousness arise in human babies? *Scientific American, 20*(5), 20–21.

Kohonen, T. (1984). Self organization and associative memory. Berlin: Springer Verlag.

Kolb, B., & Whishaw, I. Q. (1990). *Fundamentals of human neuropsychology* (3rd ed.). New York: Freeman.

Korsakoff, S. S. (1955). Psychic disorder in conjunction with peripheral neuritis (M. Victor & P. I. Yakovlev, Trans.) *Neurology, 5*, 394–406. (Original work published 1889)

Kostovic, I., & Judas, M. (2010). The development of the subplate and thalamocorticol connections in the human foetal brain. *Acta Pediatrica, 99*, 1119–1127.

Kuhl, P. K. (1991). Human adults and human infants show a "perceptual magnet effect" for the prototypes of speech categories, monkeys do not. *Perception Psychophysiology, 50*(2), 93–107.

Kuhl, P. K. (2004). Early language acquisition: Cracking the speech code. *Nature Reviews Neuroscience, 5*, 831–843.

Kuhl, P. K., & Meltzoff, A. N. (1996). Infant vocalizations in response to speech: Vocal imitation and developmental change. *Journal of the Acoustical Society of America, 100*, 2425–2438.

Kuhn, T. S. (1962). *The structure of scientific revolutions* (Vol. 2). Chicago: University of Chicago Press.

LaBar, K. S., & LeDoux, J. E. (1996). Partial disruption of fear conditioning in rats with unilateral amygdala damage: Correspondence with unilateral temporal lobectomy in humans. *Behavioral Neuroscience, 110*(5), 991–997.

LaBar, K. S., & LeDoux, J. E. (2003). Emotion and the brain: An overview. In T. E. Feinberg & M. J. Farah (Eds.), *Behavioral neurology and neuropsychology* (2nd ed., pp. 711–724). New York: McGraw-Hill Medical Publishing Division.

Lakoff, G. (1987). *Women, fire, and dangerous things: What categories reveal about the mind*. Chicago: University of Chicago Press.

Lashley, K. S. (1929). *Brain mechanisms and intelligence*. Chicago: University of Chicago Press.

Lashley, K. S. (1950). In search of the engram. In *Symposia for the Society for*

Experimental Biology (Vol. 4, pp. 2–31). Cambridge, UK: Cambridge University Press.

Lashley, K. S., & Clark, G. (1946). The cytoarchitecture of the cerebral cortex of ateles: A critical examination of architectonic studies. *Journal of Comparative Neurology, 85*(2), 223–305.

Leitao, S., Hogben, J., & Fletcher, J. (1997). Phonological processing skills in speech and language impaired children. *European Journal of Disorders of Communication, 32*(2), 91.

Lenneberg, E. H. (1967). *Biological foundations of language.* New York: Wiley.

Leonard, L. B. (1995). Phonological impairment. In P. Fletcher & B. MacWhinney (Eds.), *The handbook of child language* (pp. 573–602). Oxford, UK: Blackwell.

Lhermitte, F. (1986). Human autonomy and the frontal lobes. Part II: Patient behavior in complex and social situations: The "environmental dependency syndrome." *Annals of Neurology, 19*(4), 335–343.

Liberman, A. M., Harris, K. S., Hoffman, H. S., & Griffith, B. C. (1957). The discrimination of speech sounds within and across phoneme bounderies. *Journal of Experimental Psychology, 54*, 358–368.

Lichtheim, L. (1885). On aphasia. *Brain and Language, 7*, 433–484.

Lieberman, P. (2002). On the nature and evolution of the neural bases of human language. *American Journal of Physical Anthropology, Suppl. 35*, 36–62.

Logothetis, N. K. (1999). Vision: A window on consciousness. *Scientific American, 281*(5), 68–75.

Lumer, E. D., Friston, K. J., & Rees, G. (1998). Neural correlates of perceptual rivalry in the human brain. *Science, 280*(5371), 1930–1934.

Luria, A. (1966). *Higher cortical functions in man.* New York: Basic Books.

Maccioni, R. B., Farias, G., Morales, I., & Navarrete, L. (2010). The revitalized tau hypothesis on Alzheimer's disease. *Archives of Medical Research, 41*(3), 226–231.

Maia, T. V., & Frank, M. J. (2011). From reinforcement learning models to psychiatric and neurological disorders. *Nature Neuroscience, 14*(2), 154–162.

Mampe, B., Friederici, A. D., Christophe, A., & Wermke, K. (2009). Newborns' cry melody is shaped by their native language. *Current Biology, 19*(23), 1994–1997.

Marchman, V. A., Plunkett, K., & Goodman, J. (1997). Overregularization in English plural and past tense inflectional morphology: A response to Marcus (1995). *Journal of Child Language, 24*(3), 767–779.

Mareschal, D., Johnson, M. H., Sirois, S., Spratling, M. W., Thomas, M. S. C., & Westermann, G. (2007). *Neuroconstructivism: Vol. 1. How the brain constructs cognition.* New York: Oxford University Press.

Marie, P. (1906a). Révision de la question de l'aphasie: La troisième convolution frontalle gauche ne joue aucun rôle spéciale dans la fonction du langage. *Semaine Médicale, 21*, 241–484.

Mark, V. W., Kooistra, C. A., & Heilman, K. M. (1988). Hemispatial neglect affected by non-neglected stimuli. *Neurology, 38*(8), 1207–1211.

Markey, K. L. (1994). *The sensorimoter foundations of phonology: A computational model of early childhood articulatory and phonetic development.* Unpublished PhD dissertation, University of Colorado, Boulder, CO.

Marr, D. (1970). A theory for cerebral neocortex. *Proceedings of the Royal Society: B. Biological Sciences, 176*(1043), 161–234.

Marsh, R., Alexander, G. M., Packard, M. G., Zhu, H., & Peterson, B. S. (2005). Perceptual-motor skill learning in Gilles de la Tourette syndrome. Evidence for multiple procedural learning and memory systems. *Neuropsychologia, 43*(10), 1456–1465.

Marsh, R., Alexander, G. M., Packard, M. G., Zhu, H., Wingard, J. C., Quackenbush, G., et al. (2004). Habit learning in Tourette syndrome: A translational neuroscience approach to a developmental psychopathology. *Archives of General Psychiatry, 61*(12), 1259–1268.

Marshall, J. C. (1986). The description and interpretation of aphasic language disorder. *Neuropsychologia, 24*(1), 5–24.

Marshall, J. C., & Halligan, P. W. (1994). Left in the dark: The neglect of theory. *Neuropsychological Rehabilitation, 4*, 161–167.

Maslow, A. H. (1943). A theory of human motivation. *Psychological Review, 50*(4), 370–396.

Mathalon, D. H., Fedor, M., Faustman, W. O., Gray, M., Askari, N., & Ford, J. M. (2002). Response-monitoring dysfunction in schizophrenia: An event-related brain potential study. *Journal of Abnormal Psychology, 111*(1), 22–41.

Mayberg, H. S. (1997). Limbic-cortical dysregulation: A proposed model of depression. *Journal of Neuropsychiatry and Clinical Neuroscience, 9*(3), 471–481.

Mayberg, H. S., Lozano, A. M., Voon, V., McNeely, H. E., Seminowicz, D., Hamani, C., et al. (2005). Deep brain stimulation for treatment-resistant depression. *Neuron, 45*(5), 651–660.

McArthur, G. M., & Bishop, D. V. M. (2001). Auditory perceptual processing in people with reading and oral language impairments: Current issues and recommendations. *Dyslexia, 7*, 150–170.

McClelland, J. L., & Rumelhart, D. E. (1981). An interactive activation model of context effects in letter perception. Part 1: An account of basic findings. *Psychological Review, 88*, 375–407.

McCulloch, W. S., & Pitts, W. (1943). A logical calculus of the ideas immanent in nervous activity. *Bulletin of Mathematical Biophysics, 5*, 115–133.

McGrath, C. L., Kelley, M. E., Holtzheimer, P. E., Dunlop, B. W., Craighead, W. E., Franco, A. R., et al. (2013). Toward a neuroimaging treatment selection biomarker for major depressive disorder. *Journal of the American Medical Association Psychiatry, 70*(8), 821–829.

McGrath, L. M., Pennington, B. F., Shanahan, M. A., Santerre-Lemmon, L. E., Barnard, H. D., Willcutt, E. G., et al. (2011). A multiple deficit model of reading disability and attention-deficit/hyperactivity disorder: Searching for shared cognitive deficits. *Journal of Child Psychology and Psychiatry, 52*(5), 547–557.

McGurk, H., & MacDonald, J. (1976). Hearing lips and seeing voices. *Nature, 264*(5588), 746–748.

McKone, E., Crookes, K., Jeffery, L., & Dilks, D. D. (2012). A critical review of the development of face recognition: Experience is less important than previously believed. *Cognitive Neuropsychology, 28*(1–2), 174–212.

Meltzoff, A. N., & Moore, M. K. (1977). Imitation of facial and manual gestures by human neonates. *Science, 198*(4312), 74–78.

Menn, L., Markey, K. L., Mozer, M., & Lewis, C. (1993). Connectionist modeling and the microstructure of phonological development: A progress report. In B. de Boysson-Bardies, S. de Schonen, P. Jusczyk, P. McNeilage, & J. Morton (Eds.), *Developmental neurocognition: Speech and face processing in the first year of life* (pp. 421–433). Dordrecht, The Netherlands: Kluwer Academic Publishers.

Menon, V. (2011). Large-scale brain networks and psychopathology: A unifying triple network model. *Trends in Cognitive Sciences, 15*(10), 483–506.

Merker, B. (2007). Consciousness without a cerebral cortex: A challenge for neuroscience and medicine. *Behavioral and Brain Sciences, 30*, 63–134.

Mervis, C. B., & John, A. E. (2010). Intellectual disability syndromes. In K. O. Yeates, M. D. Ris, H. G. Taylor, & B. F. Pennington (Eds.), *Pediatric neuropsychology* (pp. 447–470). New York: Guilford Press.

Metzinger, T. (2003). *Being no one.* Cambridge, MA: MIT Press.

Metzinger, T. (2009). *The ego tunnel.* New York: Basic Books.

Miller, C. A., Kail, R., Leonard, L. B., & Tomblin, J. B. (2001). Speed of processing in children with specific language impairment. *Journal of Speech, Language, and Hearing Research, 44*(2), 416–433.

Miller, G. A. (1963). *Language and communication.* New York: McGraw Hill.

Miller, G. A. (1990). The place of language in a scientific psychology. *Psychological Science, 1,* 7.

Minsky, M., & Papert, S. (1969). *Perceptrons.* Oxford, UK: Oxford University Press.

Miyake, A., Friedman, N. P., Emerson, M. J., Witzki, A. H., Howerter, A., & Wager, T. D. (2000). The unity and diversity of executive functions and their contributions to complex "frontal lobe" tasks: A latent variable analysis. *Cognitive Psychology, 41*(1), 49–100.

Mondloch, C. J., Le Grand, R., & Maurer, D. (2003). Early visual experience is necessary for the development of some—but not all—aspects of face processing. In O. Pascalis & A. Slater (Eds.), *The development of face processing in infancy and early childhood* (pp. 99–117). Hauppauge, NY: Nova Science Publisher.

Montague, P. R., Dolan, R. J., Friston, K. J., & Dayan, P. (2012). Computational psychiatry. *Trends in Cognitive Science, 16*(1), 72–80.

Morais, J., Cary, L., Alegria, J., & Bertelson, P. (1979). Does awareness of speech as a sequence of phones arise spontaneously? *Cognition and Instruction, 7*(4), 323–331.

Morton, J., & Patterson, K. E. (1980). A new attempt at an interpretation, or, an attempt at a new interpretation. In M. Coltheart, K. E. Patterson, & J. C. Marshall (Eds.), *Deep dyslexia* (pp. 91–118). London: Routledge.

Muhlnickel, W., Elbert, T., Taub, E., & Flor, H. (1998). Reorganization of auditory cortex in tinnitus. *Proceedings of the National Academy of Sciences USA, 95*(17), 10340–10343.

Munakata, Y., McClelland, J. L., Johnson, M. H., & Siegler, R. S. (1997). Rethinking infant knowledge: Toward an adaptive process account of successes and failures in object permanence tasks. *Psychological Review, 104*(4), 686–713.

Munk, H. (1890). *Über die funktionen der grosshirnrinde.* Berlin: Hirschwald.

Murray, E. A., & Richmond, B. J. (2001). Role of perirhinal cortex in object perception, memory, and associations. *Current Opinion in Neurobiology, 11*(2), 188–193.

Nadel, L., Samsonovich, A., Ryan, L., & Moscovitch, M. (2000). Multiple trace theory of human memory: Computational, neuroimaging, and neuropsychological results. *Brain and Behavior, 10*(4), 352–368.

Naqvi, N. H., & Bechara, A. (2009). The hidden island of addiction: The insula. *Trends in Neuroscience, 32*(1), 56–67.

Nation, K. (2005). Children's reading comprehension difficulties. In M. J. Snowling & C. Hulme (Eds.), *The science of reading* (pp. 248–265). Oxford, UK: Blackwell.

Neisser, U. (1988). Five kinds of self knowledge. *Philosophical Psychology, 1*, 35–29.

Nelson, C. A. (1995). The ontogeny of human memory: A cognitive neuroscience perspective. *Developmental Psychology, 31*, 723–738.

Nemeroff, C. B. (1998). The neurobiology of depression. *Scientific American, 278*(6), 42–49.

Nestler, E. J., Hyman, S. E., & Malenka, R. C. (2009). *Molecular neuropharmacology: A foundation for clinical neuroscience* (2nd ed.). New York: McGraw Hill.

Neville, H. J., & Bavelier, D. (2002). Specificity and plasticity in neurocognitive development in humans. In M. H. Johnson, Y. Munakata, & R. Gilmore (Eds.), *Brain development and cognition: A reader* (2nd ed., pp. 251–270). Oxford, UK: Blackwell.

Neville, H. J., Coffey, S. A., Lawson, D. S., Fischer, A., Emmorey, K., & Bellugi, U. (1997). Neural systems mediating American Sign Language: Effects of sensory experience and age of acquisition. *Brain and Language, 57*(3), 285–308.

Newell, A., & Simon, H. A. (1972). *Human problem-solving*. Englewood Cliffs, NJ: Prentice-Hall.

Newell, F. N., & Bulthoff, H. H. (2002). Categorical perception of familiar objects. *Cognition, 85*(2), 113–143.

Nicolson, R. I., & Fawcett, A. J. (1990). Automaticity: A new framework for dyslexia research? *Cognition, 35*(2), 159–182.

Nicolson, R. I., Fawcett, A. J., & Dean, P. (2001). Developmental dyslexia: The cerebellar deficit hypothesis. *Trends in Neurosciences, 24*(9), 508–511.

Nittrouer, S. (1996). Discriminability and perceptual weighting of some acoustic cues to speech perception by 3-year-olds. *Journal of Speech and Hearing Research, 39*(2), 278–297.

Nittrouer, S., & Pennington, B. (2010). New approaches to the study of childhood language disorders. *Current Directions in Psychology Science, 19*(5), 308–313.

Nordahl, T. E., Carter, C. S., Salo, R. E., Kraft, L., Baldo, J., Salamat, S., et al. (2001). Anterior cingulate metabolism correlates with stroop errors in paranoid schizophrenia patients. *Neuropsychopharmacology, 25*(1), 139–148.

Nusslock, R., Almeida, J. R., Forbes, E. E., Versace, A., Frank, E., Labarbara, E. J., et al. (2012). Waiting to win: Elevated striatal and orbitofrontal cortical activity during reward anticipation in euthymic bipolar disorder adults. *Bipolar Disorders, 14*(3), 249–260.

Ohman, A. (2000). Fear and anxiety: Evolutionary, cognitive, and clinical perspectives. In M. Lewis & J. M. Haviland-Jones (Eds.), *Handbook of emotions* (2nd ed., pp. 573–593). New York: Guilford Press.

O'Keefe, J., & Nadel, L. (1978). *The hippocampus as a cognitive map*. Oxford, UK: Oxford University Press.

Olds, J., & Milner, P. (1954). Positive reinforcement produced by electrical stimulation of septal area and other regions of rat brain. *Journal of Comparative Physiology and Psychology, 47,* 419–427.

O'Reilly, R. C. (2010). The what and how of prefrontal cortical organization. *Trends in Neuroscience, 33,* 355–361.

O'Reilly, R. C., & Munakata, Y. (2000). *Computational explorations in cognitive neuroscience.* Cambridge, MA: MIT Press.

O'Reilly, R. C., Munakata, Y., Frank, M. J., Hazy, M. J., & Contributors. (2012). *Computational cognitive neuroscience* (Wiki Book, 1st ed.). Available at *http://ccnbook.colorado.edu.*

Oyama, S. (1985). *The ontogeny of information.* Cambridge, UK: Cambridge University Press.

Palminteri, S., Lebreton, M., Worbe, Y., Grabli, D., Hartmann, A., & Pessiglione, M. (2009). Pharmacological modulation of subliminal learning in Parkinson's and Tourette's syndromes. *Proceedings of the National Academy of Sciences USA, 106*(45), 19179–19184.

Panksepp, J. (1998). *Affective neuroscience: The foundations of human and animal emotions.* New York: Oxford University Press.

Panksepp, J., & Biven, L. (2012). *The archaeology of mind: Neuroevolutionary origins of human emotions.* New York: Norton.

Pascalis, O., de Schonen, S., Morton, J., Deruelle, C., & Fabre-Grenet, H. (1995). Mother's face recognition by neonates: A replication and an extension. *Infant Behavior and Development, 18,* 79–85.

Paulus, M. P., & Stein, M. B. (2006). An insular view of anxiety. *Biological Psychiatry, 60*(4), 383–387.

Pennington, B. F. (2002). *The development of psychopathology: Nature and nurture.* New York: Guilford Press.

Pennington, B. F. (2009). How neuropsychology informs our understanding of developmental disorders. *Journal of Child Psychology and Psychiatry, 50*(1–2), 72–78.

Pennington, B. F., & Bishop, D. V. M. (2009). Relations among speech, language, and reading disorders. *Annual Review of Psychology, 60,* 283–306.

Pennington, B. F., & Lefly, D. L. (2001). Early reading development in children at family risk for dyslexia. *Child Development, 72*(3), 816–833.

Perfetti, C. A., Beck, I., Bell, L. C., & Hughes, C. (1987). Phonemic knowledge and learning to read are reciprocal: A longitudinal study of first grade children. *Merrill–Palmer Quarterly, 33*(3), 283–219.

Peterson, R. L., Pennington, B. F., Shriberg, L. D., & Boada, R. (2009). What influences literacy outcome in children with speech sound disorder? *Journal of Speech, Language and Hearing Research, 52*(5), 1175–1188.

Phelps, E. A., O'Conner, K. J., Gatenby, J. C., Gore, J. C., Grillion, C., & Davis, M. (2001). Activation of the left amygdala to a cognitive representation of fear. *Nature Neuroscience, 4,* 437–441.

Pinker, S. (1995). *The language instinct.* New York: Morrow.

Pinker, S. (1999). Rules of language. *Science, 253*(5019), 530.

Plaut, D. C. (1995). Double dissociation without modularity: Evidence from connectionist neuropsychology. *Journal of Clinical and Experimental Neuropsychology, 17,* 291–321.

Plaut, D. C. (2002). Graded modality-specific specialisation in semantics: A computational account of optic aphasia. *Cognitive Neuropsychology, 19*(7), 603–639.

Plaut, D. C., & Kello, C. T. (1999). The emergence of phonology from the interplay of speech comprehension and production: A distributed connectionist approach. In B. MacWhinney (Ed.), *The emergence of language* (pp. 381–416). Mahwah, NJ: Erlbaum.

Plaut, D. C., & Shallice, T. (1993). Deep dyslexia: A case study of connectionist neuropsychology. *Cognitive Neuropsychology, 10*, 377–500.

Poldrack, R. A., Halchenko, Y. O., & Hanson, S. J. (2009). Decoding the large-scale structure of brain function by classifying mental states across individuals. *Psychological Science, 20*(11), 1364–1372.

Popper, K. R. (1959). *The logic of scientific discovery.* London: Routledge.

Posner, M. I., Walker, J. A., Friedrich, F. J., & Rafal, R. D. (1984). Effects of parietal injury on covert orienting of attention. *Journal of Neuroscience, 4*(7), 1863–1874.

Prinz, J. J. (2005). A neurofunctional theory of consciousness. In A. Brook & K. Aikins (Eds.), *Cognition and the brain: The philosophy and neuroscience movement* (pp. 381–396). New York: Cambridge University Press.

Rafal, R. D. (1997). Hemispatial neglect: Cognitive neuropsychological aspects. In T. E. Feinberg & M. J. Farah (Eds.), *Behavioral neurology and neuropsychology* (pp. 319–335). New York: McGraw-Hill.

Raichle, M. E., MacLeod, A. M., Snyder, A. Z., Powers, W. J., Gusnard, D. A., & Shulman, G. L. (2001). A default mode of brain function. *Proceedings of the National Academy of Sciences USA, 98*(2), 676–682.

Raitano, N. A., Pennington, B. F., Tunick, R. A., Boada, R., & Shriberg, L. D. (2004). Pre-literacy skills of subgroups of children with speech sound disorders. *Journal of Child Psychology and Psychiatry, 45*(4), 821–835.

Ramachandran, V. S. (2011). *The tell-tale brain.* New York: Norton.

Ramsey-Rennels, J. L., & Langlois, J. H. (2006). Infants' differential processing of female and male faces. *Current Directions in Psychological Science, 15*(2), 59–62.

Ramus, F. (2003). Developmental dyslexia: Specific phonological deficit or general sensorimotor dysfunction? *Current Opinion in Neurobiology, 13*(2), 212–218.

Rand, T. C. (1974). Letter: Dichotic release from masking for speech. *Journal of the Acoustical Society of America, 55*, 678–680.

Ranganath, C., & Blumenfeld, R. S. (2005). Doubts about double dissociations between short- and long-term memory. *Trends in Cognitive Science, 9*(8), 374–380.

Redcay, E., Haist, F., & Courchesne, E. (2008). Functional neuroimaging of speech perception during a pivotal period in language acquisition. *Developmental Science, 11*(2), 237–252.

Rice, M. L., & Wexler, K. (1996). Toward tense as a clinical marker of specific language impairment in English-speaking children. *Journal of Speech and Hearing Research, 39*(6), 1239–1257.

Rivolta, D., Palermo, R., Schmalzl, L., & Coltheart, M. (2012). Covert face recognition in congenital prosopagnosia: A group study. *Cortex, 48*(3), 344–352.

Rivolta, D., Schmalzl, L., Coltheart, M., & Palermo, R. (2011). Semantic information can facilitate covert face recognition in congenital prosopagnosia. *Journal of Clinical and Experimental Neuropsychology, 32*(9), 1002–1016.

Roberts, R. J., Jr., & Pennington, B. F. (1996). An interactive framework for examining prefrontal cognitive processes. *Developmental Neuropsychology, 12*(1), 105–126.

Rolls, E. T. (1999). *The brain and emotion.* New York: Oxford University Press.

Rosenblatt, F. (1960). *On the convergence of reinforcement procedures in simple perceptron.* New York: Cornell Aeronautical Laboratory.

Rothman, K. J., & Greenland, S. (1998). Causation and causal inference. In K. J. Rothman & S. Greenland (Eds.), *Modern epidemiology* (pp. 7–28). Philadelphia: Lippcott-Raven.

Rovee-Collier, C., & Cuevas, K. (2009). Multiple memory systems are unnecessary to account for infant memory development: An ecological model. *Developmental Psychology, 45*(1), 160–174.

Roy, M., Shohamy, D., & Wager, T. D. (2012). Ventromedial prefrontal–subcortical systems and the generation of affective meaning. *Trends in Cognitive Science, 16*(3), 147–156.

Rumelhart, D. E., & McClelland, J. L. (1982). An interactive activation model of context effects in letter perception: Part 2. The contextual enhancement effect and some tests and extensions of the model. *Psychological Review, 89,* 60–94.

Rumelhart, D. E., McClelland, J. L., & the PDP Research Group. (1986). *Parallel distributed processing: Vol. 1. Foundations.* Cambridge, MA: MIT Press.

Rutter, M. (2006). *Genes and behavior.* Malden, MA: Blackwell Publishing.

Sabatinelli, D., Bradley, M. M., Lang, P. J., Costa, V. D., & Versace, F. (2007). Pleasure rather than salience activates human nucleus accumbens and medial prefrontal cortex. *Journal of Neurophysiology, 98*(3), 1374–1379.

Sacks, O. (1973). *Awakenings.* Garden City, NY: Doubleday.

Sacks, O. (1985). *The man who mistook his wife for a hat.* New York: Summit Books.

Saffran, E. M., Aslin, R. N., & Newport, E. L. (1996). Statistical learning by 8-month-old infants. *Science, 274*(5294), 1926–1928.

Saffran, J. R. (2003). Statistical language learning: Mechanisms and constraints. *Current Directions in Psychological Science, 12*(4), 110.

Saffran, J. R., Johnson, E. K., Aslin, R. N., & Newport, E. L. (1999). Statistical learning of tone sequences by human infants and adults. *Cognition, 70*(1), 27–52.

Sams, M., Hari, R., Rif, J., & Knuutila, J. (1993). The human auditory sensory memory trace persists about 10 sec: Neuromagnetic evidence. *Journal of Cognitive Neuroscience, 5,* 363–370.

Sander, L. W. (1964). Adaptive relationships in early mother–child interaction. *Journal of the American Academy of Child Psychiatry, 3,* 231–264.

Sanders, L. (2012). Emblems of awareness. *Science News, 181*(3), 22.

Sanders, S. J., Ercan-Sencicek, A. G., Hus, V., Luo, R., Murtha, M. T., Moreno-De-Luca, D., et al. (2011). Multiple recurrent de novo cnvs, including duplications of the 7q11.23 Williams syndrome region, are strongly associated with autism. *Neuron, 70*(5), 863–885.

Scarborough, H. S. (1990). Very early language deficits in dyslexic children. *Child Development, 61*(6), 1728–1743.

Scarborough, H. S., & Parker, J. D. (2003). Children's learning and teachers' expectations: Matthew effects in children with learning disabilities: Development of reading, IQ, and psychosocial problems from grade 2 to grade 8. *Annals of Dyslexia, 53,* 47–71.

Schacter, D. L., Addis, D. R., & Buckner, R. L. (2007). Remembering the past to imagine the future: The prospective brain. *Nature Reviews Neuroscience, 8,* 657–661.

Schacter, D. L., Addis, D. R., & Buckner, R. L. (2008). Episodic simulation of future events: Concepts, data and application. *Annals of the New York Academy of Sciences, Special Issue: The Year in Cognitive Neuroscience, 1124,* 39–60.

Schacter, D. L., & Moscovitch, M. (1984). Infants, amnesic, and dissociable memory systems. In M. Moscovitch (Ed.), *Infant memory* (pp. 173–216). New York: Plenum Press.

Scherf, K. S., Behrmann, M., Humphreys, K., & Luna, B. (2007). Visual category-selectivity for faces, places and objects emerges along different developmental trajectories. *Developmental Science, 10*(4), F15–F30.

Schneider, K. (1959). *Clinical psychopathology* (5th ed.). Oxford, UK: Grune & Stratton.

Schultz, R. T. (2005). Developmental deficits in social perception in autism: The role of the amygdala and fusiform face area. *International Journal of Developmental Neuroscience, 23*(2), 125.

Schwartz, M. F. (1984). What the classical aphasia categories can't do for us, and why. *Brain and Language, 21,* 3–8.

Serniclaes, W., Van Heghe, S., Mousty, P., Carre, R., & Sprenger-Charolles, L. (2004). Allophonic mode of speech perception in dyslexia. *Journal of Experimental Child Psychology, 87*(4), 336–361.

Seymour, P. H., & Elder, E. (1986). Beginning reading without phonology. *Cognitive Neuropsychology, 3,* 1–36.

Shallice, T. (1979). Case study approach in neuropsychological research. *Journal of Clinical Neuropsychology, 1,* 183–211.

Shallice, T. (1988). *From neuropsychology to mental structure.* New York: Cambridge University Press.

Shallice, T., & Warrington, E. K. (1969). Independent functioning of verbal memory stores: A neuropsychological study. *Quarterly Journal of Experimental Psychology, 22,* 261–273.

Shanahan, M. A., Pennington, B. F., & Willcutt, E. W. (2008). Do motivational incentives reduce the inhibition deficit in ADHD? *Developmental Neuropsychology, 33*(2), 137–159.

Shankweiler, D. P., Liberman, I. Y., Mark, L. S., Fowler, C. A., & Fischer, F. W. (1979). The speech code and learning to read. *Journal of Experimental Psychology: Human Learning and Memory, 5,* 531–545.

Shatz, C. J. (1992). The developing brain. *Scientific American, 267*(3), 60–67.

Shewmon, D. A., Holmes, G. L., & Byrne, P. A. (1999). Consciousness in congenitally decorticate children: Developmental vegetative state as self-fulfilling prophecy. *Developmental Medicine and Child Neurology, 41*(6), 364–374.

Shriberg, L. D., Tomblin, J. B., & McSweeny, J. L. (1999). Prevalence of speech delay in 6-year-old children and comorbidity with language impairment. *Journal of Speech Language and Hearing Research, 42*(6), 1461–1481.

Siegelmann, H. T. (1999). *Neural networks and analog computation: Beyond the Turing limit*. Boston: Birkhauser.

Singer, W., & Gray, C. M. (1995). Visual feature integration and the temporal correlation hypothesis. *Annual Review of Neuroscience, 18*, 555–586.

Sitton, M., Mozer, M. C., & Farah, M. J. (2000). Superadditive effects of multiple lesions in a connectionist architecture: Implications for the neuropsychology of optic aphasia. *Psychological Review, 107*(4), 709–734.

Skinner, B. F. (1957). *Verbal behavior*. New York: Appleton-Century-Crofts.

Smith, E. E., & Jonides, J. (1999). Storage and executive processes in the frontal lobes. *Science, 283*(5408), 1657–1661.

Smolensky, M. H., & D'Alonzo, G. E. (1988). Biologic rhythms and medicine. *American Journal of Medicine, 85*(1B), 34–46.

Sperry, R. W. (1950). Neural basis of the spontaneous optokinetic response produced by visual inversion. *Journal of Comparative Physiological Psychology, 43*(6), 482–489.

Sporns, O., & Zwi, J. D. (2004). The small world of the cerebral cortex. *Neuroinformatics, 2*(2), 145–162.

Squire, L. R. (1987). *Memory and brain*. New York: Oxford University Press.

Stanovich, K. E. (1986). Matthew effects in reading: Some consequences of individual differences in the acquisition of literacy. *Reading Research Quarterly, 21*(4), 360–406.

Stern, D. N. (1985). *The interpersonal world of the infant: A view from psychoanalysis and developmental psychology*. New York: Basic Books.

Stuber, G. D., Britt, J. P., & Bonci, A. (2011). Optogenetic modulation of neural circuits that underlie reward seeking. *Biological Psychiatry, 71*(12), 1061–1067.

Sullivan, P. F., Daly, M. J., & O'Donovan, M. (2012). Genetic architectures of psychiatric disorders: The emerging picture and its implications. *National Review of Genetics, 13*(8), 537–551.

Swan, D., & Goswami, U. (1997a). Phonological awareness deficits in developmental dyslexia and the phonological representations hypothesis. *Journal of Experimental Child Psychology, 66*(1), 18–41.

Swan, D., & Goswami, U. (1997b). Picture naming deficits in developmental dyslexia: The phonological representations hypothesis. *Brain and Language, 56*(3), 334–353.

Tallal, P. (1980). Auditory temporal perception, phonics, and reading disabilities in children. *Brain and Language, 9*(2), 182–198.

Tallal, P. (2004). Improving language and literacy is a matter of time. *Nature Reviews Neuroscience, 5*(9), 721–728.

Tallal, P., & Piercy, M. (1973). Developmental aphasia: Impaired rate of nonverbal processing as a function of sensory modality. *Neuropsychologia, 11*, 389–398.

Talland, G. (1965). *Deranged memory*. New York: Academic Press.

Tekin, S., & Cummings, J. L. (2003). Hallucinations and related conditions. In K. M. Heilman & E. Valenstein (Eds.), *Clinical neuropsychology* (4th ed., pp. 479–494). New York: Oxford University Press.

Temple, C. M. (1988). Red is read but eye is blue: A case study of developmental dyslexia and follow-up report. *Brain and Language, 34*(1), 130–137.

Teuber, H. L. (1955). Physiological psychology. *Annual Review of Psychology, 6,* 267–296.

Thatcher, R. W. (1992). Cyclic cortical reorganization during early childhood. Special issue: The role of frontal lobe maturation in cognitive and social development. *Brain and Cognition, 20,* 24–50.

Thomas, K. M., & Nelson, C. A. (2001). Serial reaction time learning in preschool- and school-age children. *Journal of Experimental Child Psychology, 79*(4), 364–387.

Thompson, N. M., Ewing-Cobbs, L., Fletcher, J. M., Miner, M. E., & Levin, H. S. (1991). Left unilateral neglect in a preschool child. *Developmental Medicine and Child Neurology, 33,* 636–644.

Tolman, E. C. (1948). Cognitive maps in rats and men. *Psychological Reviews, 55*(4), 189–208.

Tomasello, M., & Kaminski, J. (2009). Behavior. Like infant, like dog. *Science, 325*(5945), 1213–1214.

Tomblin, J. B., Hardy, J. C., & Hein, H. A. (1991). Predicting poor communication status in preschool children using risk factors present at birth. *Journal of Speech and Hearing Research, 34*(5), 1096–1105.

Tomblin, J. B., Records, N. L., Buckwalter, P., Zhang, X., Smith, E., & O'Brien, M. (1997). Prevalence of specific language impairment in kindergarten children. *Journal of Speech, Language, and Hearing Research, 40*(6), 1245–1260.

Tononi, G. (2004). An information integration theory of consciousness. *BMC Neuroscience, 5,* 42–72.

Trauner, D., Wulfeck, B., Tallal, P., & Hesselink, J. (2000). Neurological and MRI profiles of children with developmental language impairment. *Developmental Medicine and Child Neurology, 42*(7), 470–475.

Treiman, R., Pennington, B. F., Shriberg, L. D., & Boada, R. (2008). Which children benefit from letter names in learning letter sounds? *Cognition, 106*(3), 1322–1338.

Tulving, E. (1972). Episodic and semantic memory. In E. Tulving & W. Donaldson (Eds.), *Organization of memory* (pp. 381–403). New York: Academic Press.

Tulving, E. (1985). Memory and consciousness. *Canadian Psychology, 26,* 1–12.

Ullman, M. T., & Pierpont, E. I. (2005). Specific language impairment is not specific to language: The procedural deficit hypothesis. *Cortex, 41*(3), 399–433.

Urosevic, S., Abramson, L. Y., Harmon-Jones, E., & Alloy, L. B. (2008). Dysregulation of the behavioral approach system (BAS) in bipolar spectrum disorders: Review of theory and evidence. *Clinical Psychology Reviews, 28*(7), 1188–1205.

van den Heuvel, M. P., Stam, C. J., Kahn, R. S., & Hulshoff Pol, H. E. (2009). Efficiency of functional brain networks and intellectual performance. *Journal of Neuroscience, 29*(23), 7619–7624.

van der Lely, H. K. (1994). Canonical linking rules: Forward versus reverse linking in normally developing and specifically language-impaired children. *Cognition, 51*(1), 29–72.

Van Orden, G. C., Pennington, B. F., & Stone, G. O. (1990). Word identification in reading and the promise of subsymbolic psycholinguistics. *Psychological Review, 97*(4), 488–522.

Van Orden, G. C., Pennington, B. F., & Stone, G. O. (2001). What do double dissociations prove? *Cognitive Science, 25*, 111–172.

Vargha-Khadem, F., Gadian, D. G., Watkins, K. E., Connelly, A., Van Paesschen, W., & Mishkin, M. (1997). Differential effects of early hippocampal pathology on episodic and semantic memory. *Science, 277*(5324), 376–380.

Velleman, S. L., & Mervis, C. B. (2011). Children with 7q11.23 duplication syndrome: Speech, language, cognitive, and behavioral characteristics and their implications for intervention. *Perspectives in Language and Learning Education, 18*(3), 108–116.

Vigneau, M., Beaucousin, V., Herve, P. Y., Duffau, H., Crivello, F., Houde, O., et al. (2006). Meta-analyzing left hemisphere language areas: Phonology, semantics, and sentence processing. *Neuroimage, 30*(4), 1414–1432.

Volkow, N. D., Fowler, J. S., Ding, Y. S., Wang, G. J., & Gatley, S. J. (1999). Imaging the neurochemistry of nicotine actions: Studies with positron emission tomography. *Nicotine Tobacco Research, 1*(Suppl. 2), S127–S132; discussion S139–S140.

von Helmholtz, H. (1867). *Handbuch der physiologischen optik* (1st ed.). Hamburg, Germany: Voss.

Von Holst, E. (1954). Relations between the central nervous system and the peripheral organs. *British Journal of Animal Behavior, 2*, 89–94.

Vygotsky, L. S. (1979). *Mind in society: The development of high mental processes*. Cambridge, MA: Harvard University Press.

Wagner, R. K., Torgesen, J. K., & Rashotte, C. A. (1994). Development of reading-related phonological processing abilities: New evidence of bidirectional causality from a latent variable longitudinal study. *Developmental Psychology, 30*(1), 73–87.

Walley, A. C. (1993). The role of vocabulary development in children's spoken word recognition and segmentation ability. *Developmental Review, 13*, 286–350.

Wang, L., Hosakere, M., Trein, J. C., Miller, A., Ratnanather, J. T., Barch, D. M., et al. (2007). Abnormalities of cingulate gyrus neuroanatomy in schizophrenia. *Schizophrenia Research, 93*(1–3), 66–78.

Warren, R. M. (1961). Verbal transformation and auditory perceptual mechanisms. *British Journal of Psychology, 52*, 249–258.

Wegner, D. M. (2002). *The illusion of conscious will*. Cambridge, MA: MIT Press.

Weiskrantz, L. (1968). Some traps and pontifications. In L. Weiskrantz (Ed.), *Analysis of behavioral change* (pp. 415–429). New York: Harper & Row.

Weiskrantz, L. (1986). *Blindsight: A case study and implications*. Oxford, UK: Oxford University Press.

Werbos, P. (1974). *Beyond regression: New tools for prediction and analysis in the behavioral sciences*. Cambridge, MA: Harvard University Press.

Werker, J. F., & Tees, R. C. (1984). Cross-language speech perception: Evidence for perceptual reorganization during the first year of life. *Infant Behavior and Development, 7*, 49–63.

Wernicke, C. (1874). *Der aphasische symptomenkomplex. Eine psychologische studie auf anatomischer basis*. Breslau, Germany: M. Cohn und Weigart.

Westermann, G., & Miranda, E. R. (2004). A new model of sensorimotor coupling in the development of speech. *Brain and Language, 89*, 393–400.

Whalen, P. J., Rauch, S. L., Etcoff, N. L., McInerney, S. C., Lee, M. B., & Jenike, M. A. (1998). Masked presentations of emotional facial expressions modulate amygdala activity without explicit knowledge. *Journal of Neuroscience, 18*(1), 411–418.

Whitehead, A. N., & Russell, B. (1912). *Principia mathematica* (Vol. 2). London: Cambridge University Press.

Whitfield-Gabrieli, S., & Ford, J. M. (2012). Default mode network activity and connectivity in psychopathology. *Annual Review of Clinical Psychology, 8*, 49–76.

Widrow, B., & Hoff, M. E. (1960). Adaptive switching circuits. *IRE WESCON Convention Record. Part 4: Computers: Man-Machine Systems* (96-104). New York: IRE.

Willshaw, D. J. (1972). A simple network capable of inductive generalization. *Proceedings of the Royal Society: B. Biological Science, 182*(67), 233–247.

Wilson, E. O. (1998). *Consilience: The unity of knowledge.* New York: Vintage Books.

Witthoft, N., & Winawer, J. (2013). Learning, memory, and synesthesia. *Psychological Science, 24*(3), 258–265.

Wolfe, T. (2000). *O lost: A story of the buried life.* Columbia, SC: University of South Carolina Press.

Wood, C. C. (1978). Variations on a theme of Lashley: Lesion experiments of the neuronal model of Anderson, Silverstein, Ritz & Jones. *Psychological Review, 85*, 582–591.

Wood, C. C. (1982). Implications of simulated lesion experiments for the interpretation of lesions in real nervous systems. In M. A. Arbib, D. Caplan, & J. C. Marshall (Eds.), *Neural models of language processes* (pp. 485–506). New York: Academic Press.

Yin, R. K. (1970). Face recognition by brain-injured patients: A dissociable ability? *Neuropsychologia, 8*(4), 395–402.

Young, R. M. (1970). *Mind, brain, and adaptation in the nineteenth century.* Oxford, UK: Clarendon Press.

Zeki, S. (1992). The visual image in mind and brain. *Scientific American, 267*(3), 68–76.

Zimmer, C. (2004). *Soul made flesh: The discovery of the brain and how it changed the world.* New York: Free Press.

Zola-Morgan, S., Squire, L. R., & Amaral, D. G. (1986). Human amnesia and the medial temporal region: Enduring memory impairment following a bilateral lesion limited to field CA1 of the hippocampus. *Journal of Neuroscience, 6*(10), 2950–2967.

Index

An *f* following a page number indicates a figure;
a *t* following a page number indicates a table;
page numbers in bold refer to terms in the glossary.

38 63